AF752185

Consideration of Alternative Licensing Procedures for Vaccines for Minor Species, Minor Indications and Autogenous/Autologous Products

Developments in Biologicals

Vol. 117

This series «Developments in Biologicals» begins with Vol. 102 and is the continuation of IABS symposia series «Progress in Immunobiological Standardization», Vols 1-5, «Immunobiological Standardization», Vols 1-22 and «Developments in Biological Standardization», Vols 23-101.

Organized and published by the International Association for Biologicals (IABs)

KARGER

Basel · Freiburg · Paris · London · New York ·
Bangalore · Bangkok · Singapore · Tokyo · Sydney

Consideration of Alternative Licensing Procedures for Vaccines for Minor Species, Minor Indications and Autogenous/Autologous Products

PEI Lecture Hall, Langen, Germany
October 29 – 31, 2003

Volume editor *Carmen Jungbäck*
Paul-Ehrlich-Institut, Langen, Germany

Proceedings of a meeting organized by the
International Association for Biologicals (IABs), and the
Paul-Ehrlich-Institut (PEI)

11 figures and 25 tables, 2004

KARGER Basel · Freiburg · Paris · London · New York ·
Bangalore · Bangkok · Singapore · Tokyo · Sydney

Developments in Biologicals

Bibliographic Indices. This publication is listed in bibliographic services, including Current Contents® and Index Medicus.

Drug dosage. The authors and the publisher have exerted every effort to ensure that drug selection and dosage set forth in this text are in accord with current recommendations and practice at the time of publication. However, in view of ongoing research, changes in government regulations, and the constant flow of information relating to drug therapy and drug reactions, the reader is urged to check the package insert for each drug for any change in indications and dosage and for added warnings and precautions. This is particularly important when the recommended agent is a new and/or infrequently employed drug.

Printed in Switzerland by Médecine et Hygiène, Genève.
ISBN 3-8055-7737-0

Programme Committee

David Espeseth, IABs, Perkasie, PA, USA
Daniel Gaudry, IABs, Nokomis, FL, USA
Rick E. Hill, CVB, Ames, IA, USA
Carmen Jungbäck, PEI, Langen, Germany
Philippe Vannier, AFSSA, Ploufragan, France

Organisation of the Meeting

Opening Speech

Session I	**Autogenous/Autologous Vaccines**
Session I (Part 1)	Legal Basis and Definitions: Views from Authorities, Field and Industry Moderator: *Carmen Jungbäck* (PEI)
Session I (Part 2)	Identification of Suitable and Needed Antigens and Criteria for Quality of Production and Control Moderator: *Richard Hill* (CVB, USDA, APHIS)
Session I (Part 3)	Actual Situation and Handling in the Field: Producers' and Users' Point of View Moderator: *Brigitte Bönisch* (Merial)
Session II	**Vaccine for Minor Use and Minor Species**
Session II (Part 1)	Introduction, Producers' and Veterinarians' Point of View Moderators: *David Mackay* (Laboratory Institute for Animal Health) *René Aerts* (Intervet International)
Session II (Part 2)	Necessary Changes in Legal Provisions Moderator: *Peter Jones* (EMEA)
Session II (Part 3)	Legal Basis, Definitions, Need for Availability and the Role of Conditional Licences: Authorities' Point of View Moderator: *Manfred Moos* (PEI)

Contents

Session II (Part 3)

Vaccines for Minor Use and Minor Species

Jungbäck C (ed): Consideration of Alternative Licensing Procedures for Vaccines for Minor Species, Minor Indications and Autogenous/Autologous Products.
Dev Biol. Basel, Karger, 2004, vol 117, p 1.

Opening Speech

Jungbäck C (ed): Consideration of Alternative Licensing Procedures for Vaccines for Minor Species, Minor Indications and Autogenous/Autologous Products.
Dev Biol. Basel, Karger, 2004, vol 117, pp 3-6.

Opportunities and Expectations

D.A. Espeseth

IABs, Perkasie, PA, USA

Introduction

The International Association for Biologicals (IABs) and Paul-Ehrlich-Institut (PEI) are pleased to be co-sponsors of this international veterinary meeting for consideration of alternative licensing procedures for vaccines for minor species, minor indications and autogenous/autologous products. As the title suggests, this meeting is intended to address alternative licensing procedures for these vaccines. However, we should interpret licensing procedures in the broad sense. That is, we should discuss all regulatory requirements for vaccines for minor species, minor indications and autogenous/autologous products and how they could be constructed or amended to maintain appropriate standards of purity, safety, potency, and efficacy yet provide procedures that permit or encourage the development and marketing of these products.

Issues for Consideration

Regulatory authorities are continually challenged with the task of establishing standards for veterinary vaccines that ensure appropriate levels of purity, safety, potency and efficacy, yet are not so demanding that they inhibit product availability. They have been successful in their development of such standards for vaccines for major species where potential markets are large, but have not had the same success for vaccines for minor species or minor indications where potential markets are small. The cost of complying with regulatory requirements for licensing or registration of small market vaccines is high compared to potential sales, and thus commercial companies that must make a profit to stay in business are reluctant to develop such products. As a result, many vaccines needed for use in minor species or for minor indications are not available.

Regulatory requirements for autogenous/autologous vaccines are also being considered at this meeting. Autogenous/autologous vaccines are inactivated products that are prepared from pathogenic micro-organisms isolated from an infected herd or flock for use in the immunization of animals in that herd or flock. These vaccines are often used when no suitable authorized traditional vaccine is available, such as: (i) for emerging new diseases; (ii) for disease due to emerging new strains, serotypes, or biotypes of micro-organisms that are not contained in traditional vaccines; or (iii) for diseases in minor species or for minor indications where suitable vaccines have not been developed.

Although available in Member States for use in emergency situations, harmonized regulatory requirements for the production and control of autogenous/autologous products have not been established in the European Union (E.U.). In the United States (U.S.), standards and procedures for production and control have been established, but are still controversial in regard to the controls that have been applied. In the U.S. some vaccine manufacturers have suggested that current regulations could be modified to allow more efficient use of these products without compromising prudent control. However, other vaccine manufacturers have raised concerns that some biologicals manufacturers may be abusing current regulations to bypass potency and efficacy standards in the marketing of vaccines [1].

Aim of the Meeting

This meeting provides a forum for regulatory authorities, biologicals manufacturers, representatives from animal industry, practising veterinarians, and other interested parties from the U.S. and the E.U. to exchange information and discuss regulatory and field experiences on the use and regulation of vaccines for minor species, minor indications and autogenous/autologous products. We have an opportunity in this forum to have an impact on the rules and regulations for the use of these products. As we consider the issues surrounding these products, we should try to focus on what is needed for the protection and improvement of animal health.

A reliable supply of pure, safe, potent, and effective veterinary biological products is essential for safeguarding animal health and the successful operation of animal disease control and eradication programmes. Immunization is the primary means of control for many animal diseases [2]. In the case of diseases in minor species, and diseases that have a very low prevalence in major species (minor indications), many needed products are not available. In the interest of protecting and improving animal health we need to determine how to facilitate the production of vaccines to meet these needs. We will have the opportunity to develop recommendations for new and creative approaches to resolve this problem in our round table discussions.

In our discussions and development of recommendations, we should also review these issues and the impacts of proposed solutions by applying risk analysis models used in the licensing or registration of veterinary vaccines. Risk assessment should identify any new or increased risk related to a proposed action; that is, the likelihood of an adverse event occurring and the consequences if that adverse event occurs. Risk management should approve or reject the action or apply controls or restrictions to mitigate the risks when applicable. For example, in the case of autogenous products in the US, current regulations mitigate risks by restricting production to killed products and limiting the distribution of the product to the herd of origin or other adjacent or non-adjacent herds that can be demonstrated to be at risk from the same infectious disease. We also need to apply risk communication to validate recommended actions concerning these products through a peer review process.

Availability of Products

Animal health and biologicals regulatory authorities have recognized the lack of authorized vaccines for minor species and minor indications to be a significant animal health problem [3]. They have also recognized that there are other situations in major species where no suitable traditional vaccines are available. In their efforts to address these needs, authorities in the U.S. have developed a variety of regulatory options to facilitate the availability of products such as: (i) conditional licensing, based on purity, safety, and a reasonable expectation of efficacy to meet an emergency condition, a limited market or local situation, or other special circumstance; (ii) licensing of autogenous products; (iii) authorization of production and shipment of unlicensed products for experimental use in animals or the importation of products under permit for research and evaluation; (iv) State licensing of products for administration solely within the State of production; (v) exemptions from licensing for production of biologicals by a person, firm, or corporation solely for administration to their own animals or solely for administration to animals under a veterinarian-client-patient relationship in the course of a State-licensed professional practice of veterinary medicine or for products used by the Department of Agriculture in the prevention, control, or eradication of animal disease; and (vi) permitting extra label use of vaccines by licensed Veterinarians under a Veterinarian-client patient relationship [4].

Authorities in the E.U. have also developed regulations to address these needs such as: (i) Regulation 2309/93 and Directive 2001/81/EC which permit provisional marketing authorizations to be issued when no suitable authorized medicine is available to treat a disease; (ii) special treatment authorizations may be issued in most Member States under Directive 2001/82/EEC, Article 10, for importation of products approved in another country for treatment of specific animals when no suitable authorized product is available; (iii) Directive 2001/82/EEC, Article 10 also permits Member States, in exceptional circumstances, to allow extra label use of veterinary vaccines or the use of human vaccines when an authorized veterinary vaccine is not available, and (iv) autogenous/autologous vaccines are also permitted in E.U. Member States. However, the requirements and procedures for use of these options have not been harmonized within the E.U. [3,5].

In spite of these efforts, we only have a limited number of authorized veterinary vaccines available for the prevention, or treatment of diseases of minor species and for minor indications.

Expectations from Speakers and Final Discussions

Over the next two and a half days, experts from the U.S. and the E.U. will have the opportunity to exchange information concerning their experiences and knowledge in a discussion on the availability, need, and regulation of autogenous/

autologous products and products for minor species and minor indications. The first part of the meeting will be focused on autogenous/autologous products and the second part will be applied to the discussion of products for minor species and minor indications. Regulatory authorities will review the legal basis for the regulation of these products and the rationale for the controls that are being applied or considered. Strengths and weaknesses of current or proposed regulations will be discussed and possible options for improvement presented. Veterinarians will present their views on the changing needs of veterinary practice, and the role they see for autogenous/autologous products in meeting these needs. Their thoughts on what represents good veterinary practice in the use of such products will also be valuable. Biologicals manufacturers will present standards for the production and use of autogenous/autologous products, the rationale for their use, and the procedures that are applied to ensure quality. They will address how current controls could be improved to make the use of these vaccines more efficient and how inappropriate uses could be prevented. They will also present their views on what can be done to encourage the development of vaccines for minor species and minor indications. Representatives from the animal industry will present what is actually happening in the field, how their industry and needs are changing, and their thoughts concerning the standards and controls that should be applied to these products.

Following the exchange of information on each of these topics, we will have a round table discussion session where members of the audience will be encouraged to interact on issues with a panel of the speakers. From the open exchange in these round table sessions, it is expected that recommendations will be developed that will provide guidance to regulatory authorities in their drafting, updating, or amending of requirements for these products. Hopefully we will do our jobs well and regulatory authorities will find these recommendations helpful in their efforts to find new ways to facilitate the development and availability of high quality vaccines that are needed for the protection and improvement of animal health.

References

1 Smith J: Poultry Industry Needs in Relation to Autogenous Biologics. Discussion Document USAHA Meeting 2002. Unpublished.

2 Espeseth D: Principles of veterinary vaccine production. OIE Manual for Diagnostic Tests and Vaccines. Office International Des Epizooties, 2001, pp 42-51.

3 Committee For Veterinary Medicinal Products: Position paper regarding availability of products for minor uses and minor species (MUMS). The European Agency for the Evaluation of Medicinal Products Veterinary Medicines and Inspections, 2003, Consultation 477.

4 United States Department of Agriculture: Code of Federal Regulations, Title 9, Parts 101-124. US Government Printing Office, Washington D.C., USA. 2003.

5 Committee For Veterinary Medicinal Products: Points to consider regarding efficacy requirements for minor species and minor indications. The European Agency for the Evaluation of Medicinal Products Veterinary Medicines and Inspections, 2001, Consultation 610.

Dr. D.A. Espeseth, IABs, 404 Long Leaf Dr., Perkasie, PA 18944, USA.
E-mail: daespeseth@comcast.net

Jungbäck C (ed): Consideration of Alternative Licensing Procedures for Vaccines for Minor Species, Minor Indications and Autogenous/Autologous Products.
Dev Biol. Basel, Karger, 2004, vol 117, p 7.

SESSION I (Part 1)

Autogenous/Autologous Vaccines

Legal Basis and Definitions: Views from Authorities, Field and Industry

Moderator: *C. Jungbäck* (PEI)

Jungbäck C (ed): Consideration of Alternative Licensing Procedures for Vaccines for Minor Species, Minor Indications and Autogenous/Autologous Products.
Dev Biol. Basel, Karger, 2004, vol 117, pp 9-13.

Regulation of Autogenous Biologicals in the United States

C.S. Schmellik-Sandage, R.E. Hill, Jr.

Center for Veterinary Biologics, USDA, Animal and Plant Health Inspection Service, Veterinary Services, Ames, IA, USA

Key words: Veterinary, biologicals, autogenous, regulatory

Abstract: The U.S. Department of Agriculture's Center for Veterinary Biologics (CVB) is charged with protecting American agriculture. As part of this effort, CVB licenses manufacturers to produce special biologics for use in individual flocks or livestock herds afflicted by a particular microorganism. These special products, autogenous biologicals, are inactivated vaccines used by or under the direction of a veterinarian or USDA-approved specialist and are produced under a variety of special licensing requirements.

INTRODUCTION

The Virus-Serum-Toxin Act of 1913 (21 US Code 151-159) provides the legal basis for the regulation of veterinary biologicals in the United States; the United States Department of Agriculture's Center for Veterinary Biologics (CVB) has the regulatory authority for the issuance of licenses and permits for such products. The law was intended to establish standards and control the importation of products into the United States and the distribution of products interstate, assuring the purity, safety, potency, and efficacy of veterinary biological products. Administrative regulations and standards appear in Title 9, Code of Federal Regulations, Parts 101-118, with additional programme guidance found in CVB Notices, Veterinary Services Memoranda, General Licensing Considerations, and other guidance documents. Included within the scope of this authority are specialized products intended for use within an individual herd or flock under the direction of a veterinarian or other CVB-approved specialist under a veterinarian-client-patient relationship.

Basic Licensing Requirements

In the United States, both the establishment and the biological product are licensed. Basic requirements for obtaining an establishment license include submission of a complete set of blueprints and legends describing the facility, equipment and operations in accord with good manufacturing practices. A pre-license facility inspection ensures the applicant is operating the facilities as described and in a manner which ensures products are manufactured, tested, and distributed in compliance with Federal standards. At least one product qualified for licensing is required before the issuance of the establishment license.

Basic requirements for obtaining a product license include a variety of submissions from the manufacturers. A key submission is a detailed outline of production describing the method of manufacture and testing. This outline of production establishes all the requirements for culture and media, techniques and standards for growth, harvest, and inactivation of the antigen, and procedures for bottling and testing each serial. The outline of production and other licensing documents have the force of regulation and are intended to ensure that products are prepared consistently and in accord with Federal standards. Before licensing, data must be available to establish that the final product is pure, safe, potent, and effective. Product immunogenicity/efficacy is usually demonstrated in host animal vaccination/challenge studies, or in field efficacy studies and the efficacy of each label claim must be established. Field safety testing in host animals is required in a variety of locations in a large number of susceptible animals. Satisfactory production, testing, consistency, and stability of three consecutive pre-licensing serials are required before licensing. Criteria for satisfactory testing of each batch are defined in the outline of production and the regulations. The CVB conducts confirmatory testing on the pre-licensing serials.

While autogenous products meet the bulk of the required general Federal standards, some of the requirements for data, testing, and distribution differ from conventionally licensed products.

Special Requirements for Autogenous Biologicals

Autogenous products must be prepared under license in facilities approved by the USDA and must meet many of the requirements for conventional products. Each manufacturer of an autogenous biological must obtain both a license to manufacture at a specific facility (establishment license) and a license for the autogenous product. The regulations in Part 113.113 of Title 9 of the Code of Federal Regulations provide very specific special circumstances under which autogenous biologicals may be prepared. Other requirements relative to autogenous products are further defined in USDA guidance documents (Veterinary Services Memorandum No. 800.69 and Veterinary Services Memorandum No. 800.103).

Definition and basic restrictions

Autogenous biologicals are prepared from cultures of micro-organisms which have been inactivated and are non-toxic. Such products are to be used only by or under the direction of a veterinarian with a veterinarian-client-patient relationship in the herd or flock from which the micro-organism was isolated.

Micro-organisms

Micro-organisms used as seed to prepare autogenous biologicals must be isolated from sick or dead animals in the herd or flock of origin and there must be reason to believe they are the causative agent(s) of the current disease affecting such animals. Master Seed testing by the manufacturer is not required, nor is any USDA confirmatory testing of the seeds conducted. If the agent is grown in cell culture, the cell line is tested by both the manufacturer and the CVB in accord with conventional license regulations. In general, the micro-organism(s) used for the production of autogenous biologicals may not be older than 15 months from the date of isolation, or 12 months from the date of harvest of the first serial of product resulting from the micro-organism(s), whichever comes first. The use of the isolate can be extended to 24 months with the submission of supporting information by the veterinarian or approved specialist. After 24 months, if a veterinarian or approved specialist requests continued use of the product, CVB requires the manufacturer to test for antigenicity or immunogenicity in the species for which the product is intended. Micro-organisms are not to be maintained in the biologicals manufacturer's facility beyond the time they are authorized for production. It is recommended that isolates be destroyed by the facility producing the autogenous biological at the end of the maximum period for use.

Pre-license qualification

No specific product pre-licensing data are required (host animal safety or efficacy studies, pre-licensing serials, etc., as described above for conventional products).

Testing

Due to the limited distribution via trained professionals, some of the testing (efficacy and potency) requirements for autogenous biologicals are relaxed. However, the serials of product must pass the same testing for purity and safety as serials of other product codes. This includes testing of final container samples for purity and safety by a manufacturer before shipment to the producer. For the sterility test, final container samples are tested for viable bacteria and fungi. The safety tests for this type of product are generally done in mice or guinea pigs. For avian products, the safety tests are most often done in chickens. Serials of autogenous products are not tested for potency or efficacy.

Labelling

Autogenous biologicals must include a label precaution that potency and efficacy have not been established. Labelling must include the following statements: "Potency and efficacy of autogenous biologicals have not been established," and "This product is prepared for use only by or under the direction of a veterinarian under a veterinarian-client-patient relationship." No claims for duration of immunity can be made.

Serial release

The CVB allows the first serial prepared by a manufacturer to be released quickly. The first serial can be shipped after three days of satisfactory test results and the testing is then continued after shipping. (Subsequent serials will not be released under the expedited rules and will, therefore, require a longer time for delivery). If the complete series of testing after shipping is not satisfactory, manufacturers are required to recall the product.

Shipment of an autogenous biologicals serial

A manufacturer should ship autogenous biologicals serials to the veterinarian or approved specialist, unless documentation of permission to ship directly to the owner of the herd of origin has been provided. With special approval from CVB and the State Veterinarian, the product may be provided to owners of other herds.

Restrictions

Restriction to herd or flock of origin

Under normal circumstances, micro-organisms from one herd or flock must not be used to prepare a product for another herd or flock. Adjacent or non-adjacent herd or flock authorizations may be granted under certain circumstances when those herds or flocks are considered to be at risk. Specific information required for such authorizations include:

1 Name, address, and telephone number of the owner of the herd of origin.

2 Attending veterinarian's name, address, and telephone number.

3 Animal species and number in herd of origin.

4 Identification of micro-organism(s), at least to genus.

5 Diagnosis or clinical signs of the disease observed.

6 Name and address of the person who isolated the micro-organism(s) and the date of isolation.

7 Number of doses of autogenous biological requested and vaccination schedule.

8 Each adjacent herd owner's name, address, and telephone number.

9 Number of animals and species in each adjacent herd.

10 The attending veterinarian's or approved specialist's assessment of the involvement of the adjacent herd(s) with the disease observed.

Limitations on micro-organisms

All licenses for autogenous products include the restriction that the license does not authorize production, distribution, or shipment of autogenous vaccine/bacterin for foot-and-mouth disease, rinderpest, any H5 or H7 subtype of avian influenza, any subtype of avian influenza in chickens, swine vesicular disease, Newcastle disease, African swine fever, classical swine fever, *Brucella abortus*, vesicular stomatitis, rabbit haemorrhagic disease or any other disease that the USDA determines may pose a risk to animal or public health. Autogenous avian influenza vaccine may be used in turkeys but there are some additional restrictions.

Practices not recommended

- No autogenous product should be combined with other fractions or products (autogenous or commercially licensed). Interference studies have not been performed to support mixing of fractions or products.
- Micro-organisms should not be re-submitted. The growth of micro-organisms on laboratory culture can change the antigenicity of the isolate in unknown fashions.
- Mixed cultures from diagnostic laboratories should not be sent to autogenous manufacturers. Separate, pure cultures with their individual dates of isolation should be submitted to the manufacturing firm.

Summary

Vaccination is widely recognized as a valuable tool in controlling animal disease and autogenous biologicals provide an additional mechanism for veterinarians to assist consumers in maintaining healthy animals. While these products provide an additional tool in battling animal disease, autogenous biologicals are very specialized products that are prepared, tested and distributed in a manner very different from conventional vaccines. Users must be aware that these products are not prepared and tested in the same manner as traditional products and be knowledgeable of the specialized requirements before choosing to use such products.

References

1 Title 9 Code of Federal Regulations. Part 113.113 Autogenous biologics, 2003, pp 641-644.

2 Veterinary Services Memorandum 800.69. Guidelines for Autogenous Biologics. August 30, 2002.

3 Veterinary Services Memorandum 800.103. Reissuing of Product Licenses for Autogenous Products and Guidance Concerning Restrictions on the Production and Use of Veterinary Biologics. March 5, 2002.

4 Center for Veterinary Biologics Notice No. 02-04. Autogenous Vaccine Use in Turkeys.

Dr. R.E. Hill, Jr., Center for Veterinary Biologics, USDA, Animal and Plant Health Inspection Service, Veterinary Services, Suite 104, 510 South 17th Street, Ames, IA 50010, USA.
E-mail : rick.e.hill@aphis.usda.gov

Jungbäck C (ed): Consideration of Alternative Licensing Procedures for Vaccines for Minor Species, Minor Indications and Autogenous/Autologous Products.
Dev Biol. Basel, Karger, 2004, vol 117, pp 15-18.

Autogenous Vaccines: the Legal Basis and Regulation in the United Kingdom

M. Ilott

Immunologicals Team, Veterinary Medicines Directorate, Woodham Lane, New Haw, Addlestone, Surrey, KT15 3LS, United Kingdom.

Key words: Autogenous vaccines, regulation, veterinary, medicines act.

Abstract: The Veterinary Medicines Directorate is the competent authority in the U.K. for ensuring the quality, safety and efficacy of veterinary medicinal products placed on the market. The Immunologicals team is responsible for the assessment of immunological applications for Marketing Authorisations and the Inspection of manufacturing sites that produce them. In addition to these activities, the team is also responsible for the assessment of applications for emergency product licences (autogenous vaccines) and the inspection of the facilities to manufacture them. These licences authorise the manufacture of inactivated vaccines, which are manufactured from pathogens obtained from an animal or animals from a holding and used for the treatment of the animals in that holding.

Definitions

Autogenous, derives from the Greek meaning "self-produced", or originating within the body, and has a more specific meaning in relation to veterinary vaccines referring to any vaccine made from pathogens or antigens obtained from an animal or animals from a holding and used for the treatment of that animal or animals of that holding in the same locality.

Autologous derives similarly from the Greek referring to the individual organism in that it is either derived from the same individual or occurs naturally and normally in a certain tissue or structure in the body. Autologous vaccines are vaccines produced from an individual animal and used to treat that same animal i.e. papilloma vaccine derived from the animal it used to treat.

In the U.K., the preferred term for an autogenous vaccine is emergency vaccine, while autologous vaccines are not regulated by the VMD. The U.K.

Licensing Authority is prepared to consider the issue of emergency vaccine authorisations (Emergency Product Licences [EPLs]), on a one-off basis, to respond to the urgent need for a vaccine for certain disease outbreaks on a localised farm basis, where there is no U.K. licensed vaccine available for use. The scheme relates exclusively to inactivated vaccines to eliminate the possibility of spread of the vaccine strain.

Legal Basis

Directive 2001/82/EC, the community code relating to veterinary medicinal products, provides the legal basis for the regulation of these products in the European Union. Articles 3 and 4 of this Directive provide for the possibility of producing autogenous vaccines outside the regulatory framework for products issued by the marketing authorisations. Article 3 states that the Directive shall not apply to inactivated immunological veterinary medicinal products (IVMPs), which are manufactured from pathogens and antigens obtained from an animal or holding and used for the treatment of that animal or animals in the same holding in the same locality. Article 4, in contrast, gives the option to Member States to exclude from the requirements of the Directive non-inactivated IVMPS produced under the same criteria as stated under Article 3. Therefore, inactivated autogenous vaccines are outside the scope of the Directive, whereas live autogenous vaccines are within the scope, unless Member States make specific provisions to permit their use under national legislation.

Article 10 provides the basis for the prescribing cascade and it is clear that, under these provisions, a veterinary surgeon may administer an extemporaneous preparation to an animal or small number of animals where there is no authorised product and no veterinary medicinal product authorised for use in another animal species, or for another indication in the same species and where no authorised human product exists. It is not entirely clear whether or not autogenous vaccines are subject to the cascade, but in the U.K. emergency vaccines are only issued where no authorised product exists or the product has been shown to lack the expected efficacy on the holding concerned.

In the U.K., emergency product licences are issued under the 1968 Medicines Act. Article 9 exempts a veterinary surgeon from certain requirements under the act for veterinary medicinal products specially prepared for administration to a particular animal or herd under his/her care. However, the exemptions under Article 9 shall not have effect to exempt from the restrictions imposed by Articles 7 and 8 anything done by a veterinary surgeon:

(i) in relation to a vaccine specially prepared for administration to poultry;

(ii) to any other vaccine, unless the vaccines is specially prepared for administration to the animal from which it is derived;

(iii) in relation to plasma or serum, unless the plasma or serum is specially prepared for administration to one or more animals in the herd from which it is derived.

Therefore, autogenous (emergency) vaccine manufacturers in the U.K. are subject to a system of product authorisation and inspection.

Regulation of Emergency Vaccines in the United Kingdom

The emergency vaccine scheme in the U.K. has been operating since 1970.The urgent need for the vaccine shall be justified and no authorised product for the pathogen shall be available. The isolate is taken from one or more animals from a holding, but may only be used on the holding from which the isolate was made. The VMD has interpreted the term "holding" to extend to geographical sites of close proximity under certain conditions. In addition the use of an emergency vaccine at related sites, such as a holding for rearing and/or finishing may be justified under certain exceptional circumstances.

The veterinary surgeon making an application for an emergency product licence must provide details of the source and nature of the isolate, the location of the animals and the volume of vaccine required. The production method must be described, including the method of inactivation and sensitivity of the inactivation assay. The starting materials of biological origin must meet the requirements of the joint CPMP/CVMP Note for Guidance on minimising the risks of transmitting spongiform encephalopathy agents via human and veterinary medicinal products and any residue issues should be addressed. The details of the in-process and final product tests should be provided and the final product tests must include a satisfactory sterility and target species batch safety test. The target animal safety test is usually performed on two animals on the holding for where the product is intended to be used and the animals should be observed for local and systemic reactions for at least seven days before its use. The veterinary surgeon is also responsible for ensuring pharmaco-vigilance reports are submitted where necessary.

The manufacturing facilities are subject to inspection to ensure the containment of the antigen(s) and protection from cross-contamination is adequate, given the restricted use of an emergency vaccine. The inspection ensures an appropriate Quality Assurance (QA) system is in place and the equipment used in the production and quality control (QC) is properly validated. The inactivation and sterility tests are thoroughly assessed to provide adequate assurances on the appropriateness of the test methods and controls put in place by the manufacturer to minimise the risks and consequences of inadequate inactivation or non-sterile products.

Emergency Vaccines in the United Kingdom

Emergency vaccines are an important additional tool in the control and prevention of a number of animal diseases improving both the health and welfare of animals and also in protecting public health. The vaccines are limited in their potential to solve many of the availability issues surrounding minor species and minor use (MUMS) owing to the restrictions placed on their manufacture and the requirement that the products are used on the holding from which the isolate was sourced. In the U.K. emergency product licences are primarily issued for inactivated bacterial vaccines for conditions in minor species or for minor use in major species.

Emergency product licences are frequently issued to combat diseases in most domestic species and in some exotic species. In poultry, emergency vaccines have been used to treat a number of conditions including fowl cholera (*Pasteurella multocida*) in turkeys and layers, egg peritonitis in breeders and commercial layers caused by *Escherichia coli* and septicaemia in ducks due to *Reimeralla anatipestifer*. In pigs, emergency vaccines are frequently produced to treat Glasser's disease by isolating *Haemophilus parasuis* serotypes, "greasy pig disease" caused by *Staphylococcus hyicus* and septicaemia and arthritis associated with *Actinobacillus (Haempohilus) pleuropneumoniae*. In cattle a number of vaccines for papillomas have been authorised and occasional salmonella isolates have been used to treat outbreaks on a holding. In sheep there has been an increasing usage of emergency vaccines, principally due to the increasing prevalence of caseous lymphadenitis (CLA) caused by *Corynebacterium pseudotuberculosis*. This disease was introduced into the U.K. via imported goats in the 1980s and has subsequently spread rapidly to sheep and is a particular problem in certain breeds such as the Suffolk.

Conclusions

The authorisation of emergency vaccines under the 1968 Medicines act has been used successfully for over thirty years to treat a number of diseases in most domestic species and has contributed to both animal health and welfare and the protection of public health. The scheme is an important tool in the armoury of veterinarians to combat a number of diseases where there are no authorised products or where existing products and measures have failed to control an infection on a holding. Emergency vaccines do not meet the full requirements of quality, safety and efficacy as required under Directive 2001/82/EC, but the licensing authority ensures that adequate controls on the quality and safety of the products are in place to minimise the risks to both animals, the users of the products and consumers. As availability issues for minor use and minor species have become increasingly evident in Europe there is a potential for these products to fill the gap in some areas. However, owing to the restriction on the manufacture and use of the products, autogenous vaccines have only a limited poential to address many of the current issues surrounding the availability of veterinary medicines.

References

1 Directive 2001/82/EC Of The European Parliament and of the Council of 6 November 2001 on the community code relating to veterinary medicinal products.

2 Medicines Act 1968. An Act to make new provisions with respect to medicinal products and related matters, and for purposes connected therewith. (25th October 1968).

3 Committee For Proprietary Medicinal Products (CPMP), Committee For Veterinary Medicinal Products (CVMP) Note for Guidance on minimising the risks of transmitting spongiform encephalopathy agents via human and veterinary medicinal products. EMEA/410/01 rev 1. 31 May 2001.

Dr. M. Ilott, Immunologicals Team, Veterinary Medicines Directorate, Woodham Lane, New Haw, Addlestone, Surrey, KT15 3LS, United Kingdom.
E-mail: m.ilott@vmd.defra.gsi.gov.uk

Jungbäck C (ed): Consideration of Alternative Licensing Procedures for Vaccines for Minor Species, Minor Indications and Autogenous/Autologous Products.
Dev Biol. Basel, Karger, 2004, vol 117, pp 19-25.

Veterinary Autogenous Vaccines

A. Hera, J. Bures

Institute for the State Control of Veterinary Biologicals and Medicaments, Brno, Czech Republic

Abstract: Autogenous vaccines remain a regulatory issue. They are demanded by practising veterinarians and by animal owners and they are quite widely used, mainly in Central European Countries, the Czech Republic, Hungary and Slovak Republic having probably the longest tradition with these products in Central Europe. The scope given in Article 3, Para. 2 (and/or Article 4 for some countries) of Directive 2001/82/EC applies to these products in the Acceding Countries.
As these products are exempt from the harmonised regulation at the EU level, they are regulated by individual countries, the regulation varying from practically no regulatory measures in certain countries to a quite complex and demanding regulation in the other countries.
Both risks and benefits are related to these products and they shall be taken into account when regulatory measures are considered. The major risks related to veterinary autogenous vaccines relate to possibility of transmission of TSE agents or other viral, bacterial and/or fungal contaminants.
As appropriate and well balanced regulation of these products is deemed necessary, considering the risks related to these products, and based on the fact that national regulatory measures could be considered as a trade barrier under certain circumstances, harmonisation of the key issues or legal admission of the nationally based regulatory measures, including movement of these products from the other Member States, shall be laid down in the EU legislation.
The veterinary autogenous vaccines complying with basic quality and safety requirements are thus a very useful tool in the animal health and welfare management but their use should be restricted to situations where there is no authorised veterinary medicinal product available and veterinary autogenous vaccines must not be allowed to replace good farming or veterinary practices.

If we consider the issue of veterinary autogenous/autologous vaccines, we shall address three aspects related to these products. First, we must consider the necessity of having these products available on the markets – are these products important and beneficial? If we respond yes, then we should ask how important they are, and here we consider two other issues: namely what should be their position on the market and how should these products be regulated?

In order to try to give suggestion concerning these issues, we have addressed the acceding countries with a questionnaire, trying to obtain some information about the practices applied in these countries with respect to autogenous/autologous vaccines.

Based on the responces received, the practices and expectations of the ACs were summarised and suggestions concerning the future of these products are presented. As regards the importance, only three countries responded that these products are important. I feel that the importance of the autogenous/autologous vaccines cannot be understood as a number of the doses sold per year, but if we allow these products to be marketed in a country – and responses presented in the questionnaires show that these products are marketed/used in most ACs — we must be aware of the risks and benefits which the marketing and administration of these products bring.

Overview of importance of VAVs for individual ACs						
Czech Republic	Estonia	Hungary	Latvia	Poland	Slovenia	Slovakia
Yes	Yes	No	No	No	No	Yes

The most important risks which the VAVs bring are:

- the possibility of transmission of transmissive spongiform encephalopathies, which deserves special attention;
- the possibility of transmission of other extraneous agents (extraneous viral, bacterial/mycoplasma pathogens);
- the presence of live antigens/pathogens with unknown biological properties in case of lack of efficacy of the inactivation process;
- the lack of safety for the target species (toxins, endotoxins);
- the lack of efficacy (stability, adsorption of antigens to adjuvants).

Another aspect which will be considered when we address the importance of autogenous vaccines for a specified country is the availability of authorised veterinary imunologicals for given species and/or indications. Based on available information, these products are most widely used in the Central European Countries, namely in the Czech Republic, Slovak Republic and Hungary. Although the trends show progressive reduction in the use of veterinary autogenous vaccines in the Slovak Republic, they still play an important part of the animal health care in the Czech Republic and in Slovakia.

Overview of doses of veterinary autogenous vaccines marketed in the Czech Republic and in the Slovak Republic		
	Czech Republic	Slovak Republic
2000		730000
2001		250000
2002	2641765	130 000
2003 (by 31.7.2003)	1602655	40000

The autogenous vaccines are most often used in pigs and cattle (calves), poultry (particularly geese, ducks and turkey). Animals such as sheep, rabbits and dogs were reported to be target species in which the autogenous vaccines are seldom used.

Overview of target animal species in the Czech Republic	
	%
Pigs	**85**
Rabbits	**9**
Cattle	**6**

As regards the pathogens for which the VAVs are used most commonly, the figures from the Czech Republic show that the following pathogens are used most frequently:

Antigen/pathogen	%
Pasteurella multocida	**26**
Actinobacillus pleuropneumoniae	**23**
Clostridium perfringens	**10**
Escherichia coli	**10**
Bordetella bronchiseptica	**7**
Streptococcus C	**5**
Streptococcus species	**6**
Arcanobacterium pyogenes	**2**
Pasteurella haemolytica	**3**
Streptococcus porcinus	**2**

Other antigens/pathogens used less frequently are for example Moraxella bovis, Haemophilus somnus, Salmonella typhimurium and others.

Most ACs have no legislation in force which would contain provisions on veterinary autogenous vaccines. Only two countries responded that they have legislation in force regulating veterinary autogenous vaccines.

Overview of national legislation concerning veterinary autogenous vaccines						
Czech Republic	Estonia	Hungary	Latvia	Poland	Slovenia	Slovakia
Yes	No	Yes	No	No	No	No

Three countries reported that they have other regulatory instruments in place restricting certain aspects of development, manufacture, marketing or use of veterinary autogenous vaccines.

Overview of other regulatory instruments for veterinary autogenous vaccines						
Czech Republic	Estonia	Hungary	Latvia	Poland	Slovenia	Slovakia
Yes	Yes	NA	NA	No	No	Yes

As regards the possibility to have live antigens/pathogens in the veterinary autogenous vaccines, we have learned that it is not possible to find any one acceding country in which the life vaccines could be classified as veterinary autogeous vaccines.

Overview of possibility to have live antigens/pathogens in the veterinary autogenous vaccines						
Czech Republic	Estonia	Hungary	Latvia	Poland	Slovenia	Slovakia
No	No	No	NA	No	No	No

Some ACs exclude certain animal species from the species for which the veterinary autogenous vaccines can be manufactured. This applies to horses in the Czech and Slovak Republic and to poultry in the Czech Republic.

Are there any target species excluded from the veterinary autogenous vaccines?						
Czech Republic	Estonia	Hungary	Latvia	Poland	Slovenia	Slovakia
Poultry Equidae	No	No	NA	No	No	Horses

The ACs were further asked if they regulate the following areas:

- development of VAVs;
- collection of antigens for manufacture of VAVs;
- manufacture of VAVs;
- quality aspects of VAVs;
- safety aspects of VAVs;
- efficacy aspects of VAVs;
- conditions for release of the VAVs to the market;

– marketing of VAVs;
– post-marketing aspects (ADRs, quality defects reporting);
– any other aspects.

Only three countries responded that they regulate some of the areas specified above. These are Hungary regulating quality, safety and safety of VAVs, conditions for release of the VAVs into the market and postmarketing aspects, the Slovak Republic regulating the same aspects as Hungary and marketing in addition, and the Czech Republic regulating in addition to Hungary and the Slovak Republic a collection of antigens/pathogens used for the manufacture of VAVs.

Overview of regulated aspects in the ACs							
	Czech Republic	Estonia	Hungary	Latvia	Poland	Slovenia	Slovakia
development							
collection of antigens	x						
manufacture	x		x				x
quality aspects	x		x				x
safety aspects	x		x				x
efficacy aspects							
release to market conditions	x		x				x
marketing	x						x
post-marketing aspects	x		x				x
other aspects							

As I am the most familiar with the situation in the Czech Republic, I would like to give a brief description of the regulatory measures taken in this country. First it is prescribed that the manufacture of veterinary autogenous vaccines can begin only when based on the veterinary prescription of the attending veterinarian.

The manufacturer must be in possession of the manufacturing authorisation for veterinary medicinal products with the scope of the licence for veterinary immunologicals — veterinary autogenous vaccines. The manufacturer himself shall collect/process the antigens. The manufacturer is empowered to use the in-contract manufacturer/laboratory for the collection/processing of the antigens/pathogens. The manufacture must be done under the GMP conditions applicable to veterinary immunologicals – i.e. the manufacturer must comply with GMP for requirements for:

- quality assurance system;
- premises;
- personnel;
- documentation;
- production;
- quality control;
- complaint recalls;
- in-contract manufacture;
- self-inspection.

Also requirements for qualified persons apply.

There are several specific GMP provisions which the manufacturers of VAVs have to comply with. It is forbidden to manufacture live veterinary autogenous vaccines and autogenous vaccines for use in equidae and in poultry. The manufacturer must have a "standard" composition of the vaccine developed with given specifications (i.e. composition in terms of adjuvans, preservatives and other excipients used). Specifications for these compositions shall be made available to the competent authority. Any variations to these companies' specifications shall be notified to the competent authority.

The manufacturer is further obliged to sent a notification to the competent authority and to regional veterinary administration before the manufacture of a batch is started; the veterinary prescriptions constitute part of the documentation and must be kept by the manufacturers for a prescribed period and the manufacturer can use the antigens/pathogens for maximum of six months and after then he is obliged to satisfy himself that these antigens/pathogens are still applicable from the epidemiological point of view. The amount of the VAV cannot exceed the amount prescribed in the veterinary prescription.

As regards substances used in the manufacture of VAVs other than antigens/pathogens, only those substances can be used which comply with pharmacopeial standards. This is regarded as one of the most important quality aspects mainly from the point of view of minimising the risk of extraneous agents (TSEs, mycoplasmas, extraneous viruses).

The manufacture must have the inactivation process validated, and as regards inactivation, pharmacopeial criteria apply to this process. Conditions for release of VAVs into the market relate both to the quality and safety of the VAVs. Testing for microbiological quality is prescribed, meaning that the VAVs have to comply with Ph. Eur. microbial quality criteria set for veterinary immunologicals (sterility for injectables) before they are released on the market.

Next, a safety testing on the target animals must be carried out before release of the batch on to the market. The animals used for this test shall not have been vaccinated previously against the disease in question. The labelling requirements apply before the release of the batch on the market.

The VAV can be supplied only to the prescribing veterinarian and can be used only by him/her. The rules state that VAVs beyond their expiry date, or those with recognised quality defects and VAVs which were kept under other storage conditions than given by the manufacturer, cannot be used.

As regards use, the veterinary autogenous vaccines can be used only if relevant authorised VMP is not available for the disease concerned and may be used only in the herd and locality where the antigens/pathogens were collected. Before the use of the VAV in the herd, the veterinarian is obliged to carry out a safety test on the animals in the herd in accordance with the manufacturer´s instructions. As regards the postmarketing measures, both the veterinarian and the manufacturer are legally obliged to report occurrence of quality defects and adverse reactions to the VAV concerned.

If we look back on the complex issue of veterinary autogenous vaccines and if we consider the risks which may be related to the use of veterinary autogenous vaccines, it is clear that the key steps in the chain starting from preparation to use of VAVs shall be regulated to provide appropriate quality and safety of these products.

All ACs countries expressed their opinion that the EU legislation should contain provisions concerning veterinary autogenous vacines and the rules applicable to these products shall be thus harmonised at a proportionate level.

The ACs called most often for establishment of rules for:

- manufacture;
- quality and
- safety of veterinary autogeous vaccines.

This is becoming more and more important when the accession date is approaching as the basic freedoms laid down by the Treaty establishing the EU – namely free movement of goods and free movement of people and individual rights – must be observed by the EU Member States.

Setting any national restrictions with regards to trade, as with any national requirements for quality/safety of products, labelling, marketing etc. can be viewed as a barrier to trade and their implementation could be referred to the European Commission or even to the European Court of Justice. It would therefore be feasible to have the very basic conditions for these products covered by relevant EC legislation.

To solve the above-mentioned problems, the admission of national measures in the field of VAVs would be satisfactory. In conclusion the veterinary autogenous vaccines still have their place in veterinary medicine, in particular with regard to the reduced availability of authorised VMPs for minor indications and/or minor species. On the other hand, we have to consider risks related to these products, in particular the transmission of extraneous agents, the presence of which might have immense impact on animal health, consumers and, last but not least, for the credit and economic results of the farmers, veterinarians, food processing industry and of the pharmaceutical industry.

The veterinary autogenous vaccines complying with basic quality and safety requirements are a very useful tool in the animal health and welfare management but their use shall be restricted to those situations where there is no authorised veterinary medicinal product available and veterinary autogenous vaccines must not be in the position of correcting bad farming or veterinary practices.

Dr. J. Bures, Institute for the State Control of Veterinary Biologicals and Medicaments, Hudcova 56a, Brno 62100, Czech Republic.
E-mail: bures@uskvbl.cz

Jungbäck C (ed): Consideration of Alternative Licensing Procedures for Vaccines for Minor Species, Minor Indications and Autogenous/Autologous Products.
Dev Biol. Basel, Karger, 2004, vol 117, pp 27-30.

Autogenous Vaccines: Industry Proposals for Procedures and Requirements

S. Zänker

International Federation for Animal Health, Brussels, Belgium

Background

An increasing trend can be observed in veterinary practice towards the use of herd-specific vaccines, which are often being manufactured by relatively small firms and laboratories and by veterinary practices. In herds with problematic pathogens for which no commercial vaccines are available, herd-specific vaccines are often a valuable tool and will therefore continue to play an important role in the future. It is, however, necessary to minimise the associated risks for animal health and consumer protection and to avoid negative repercussions on the development and supply of safe, high-quality vaccines.

Articles 3 and 4 of Directive 2001/82/EC provide for this possibility, i.e. to produce herd-specific vaccines outside the normal legal requirements. Indeed, exemption from the requirements of the Directive are possible for:

- **inactivated** vaccines which are manufactured from pathogens and antigens obtained from an animal or animals from a holding and used for the treatment of that animal or the animals of that holding in the same locality. (Directive shall **not** apply)
- **non-inactivated** vaccines Member States **may** provide that the Directive shall not apply.

Through a survey among its members, IFAH-Europe has investigated the implementation of these provisions in the different Member States (see Annex 1). It can be noted that:

- the EU Member States handle the use and licensing of the autogenous vaccines very differently, as in fact there is no legislation in place to cover the requirements for production and control.

- IFAH-Europe believes that a more harmonised approach would be beneficial, as:
  (i) the use of non-licensed/autogenous vaccines is increasing and therefore may cause problems for proper disease control, animal health and consumer safety;
  (ii) most of the autogenous products are not really controlled as to quality, safety and efficacy, before their use;
  (iii) the use of most of these products is not really known to authorities, which is in contradiction to the pharmaco-vigilance obligations;
  (iv) this might have an impact on the overall prophylactic strategies using commercially available and fully licensed vaccines and their future development.

Requirements Regarding the Manufacture of Herd-Specific Vaccines

In most countries numerous vaccines are being produced every year for herd-specific purposes. The Paul Ehrlich Institute (PEI) in Langen has asserted (e.g. at the DVG conference on «Animal Diseases» in April 2000, Hanover) that numerous pathogens are being used for the manufacture of herd-specific vaccines in the livestock and companion animal sectors. These not only include bacterial pathogens such as Staphylococci, Streptococci, Pasteurella, E. coli, Salmonellae and Clostridia, but also various viral pathogens such as rota-, corona-, BRS and BVD viruses (!) and chlamydia. Therefore, we believe that the criteria for producing and testing of autogenous vaccines should be better defined:

- **Inactivation** tests are not mandatory in some countries, such as Germany, the U.K. and the Netherlands. No evidence of inactivation is required. There is consequently a danger of pathogenic agents being spread. In the interests of disease control it is in our view absolutely essential that the pathogen in question be safely inactivated, regardless of whether it is bacterial or viral. This is stipulated in the above-mentioned EU Directive 2001/82/EC, which exempts only inactivated immunological veterinary medicinal products in the form of autologous or herd-specific vaccines.
- Furthermore, the production of autogenous vaccines should be **limited to bacterial** vaccines. The multiplication of viral pathogens is associated with an elevated risk of contamination due to the use of cell cultures and serum additives. Exemptions may be allowed for the manufacture of herd-specific viral vaccines and should be limited to vaccines in which no multiplication in cell cultures takes place (e.g. papilloma vaccines). If viral herd-specific vaccines were considered necessary for an animal, specific requirements would have to be defined.
- Concerning the **production** of autogenous vaccines, the qualification of the person entitled to produce and control the equipment and the premises should be defined. The companies or institutions should have a manufacturing licence and should be controlled.

- **To test efficacy**, in view of the lack of time and unfeasibility to test each batch, or to run a large battery of tests, we would suggest that only a reduced data set is required to assess the activity of the vaccines, including e.g. serology tests.
- To ensure **safety**, a reduced pre-testing in a small group of animals would be recommended. A standard safety test on each batch would probably not be feasible.
- With regard to consumer protection and MRLs, it would also be necessary to rule out potential threats to animal and consumer health resulting from potential residues of vaccine adjuvants used for the purposes of inactivation and preservation (e.g. formalin). At the same time, these products should be subject to the same maximum residue limits and threshold values as are required for licensed vaccines. For preservatives such as e.g. thiomersal and timerfonate, the maximum values laid down in the Regulation on Maximum Residue Limits (Reg 2377/90/EEC) apply for all food-producing animals. No exemptions have been provided for herd-specific vaccines. Compliance with these maximum values is to be demonstrated by means of appropriate tests. Further threshold values (e.g. for formalin) as laid down in the European Pharmacopoeia (Monograph 0062 on Vaccina ad usum veterinarium) should be made mandatory.
- With regard to **stability**, due to lack of data, it is recommended that the shelf life be restricted to six months unless other data can be provided by the applicant to justify a longer shelf life.
- The provision of a test for **sterility** in accordance with the European Vaccines Monograph should also be required for herd-specific vaccines.
- Similarly, **starting material** should be in accordance with the requirements of the European Pharmacopoeia.

Requirements Regarding the Use of Herd Specific Vaccines

IFAH-Europe believes that the conditions of use should also be better clarified. First of all:

- The use of a herd specific vaccine should only be permitted in the case where no commercial vaccine is available in the country concerned. If a licensed vaccine is available in another Member State, the first choice would be to import under specific conditions ("Cascade") before an autogenous vaccine can be produced. The veterinarian in charge should take this decision.
- The extent of use, i.e. definition of a "herd", should also be clarified. IFAH-Europe believes that the use of a herd-specific vaccine should be restricted to the herd where the agent was isolated from, in accordance with EU legislation
- The use of autogenous vaccines or, alternatively, imported vaccines, should also be controlled for reasons of pharmaco-vigilance, to be able to trace any potential adverse reaction.

Repercussions on the Market Due to Distortion of Competition

In most countries, herd-specific vaccines are not required to meet the same quality and safety requirements as commercially produced vaccines. They are therefore considerably less costly to manufacture and are also increasingly being used where commercial vaccines are available. Besides the distortion of competition and the discrimination against manufacturers of commercial vaccines, the development of new vaccines (e.g. for circo viruses) is also being threatened due to a lack of incentives for companies.

One frequently-stated advantage of herd-specific vaccines is their rapid availability due to the less stringent development and manufacturing requirements. In some cases, the interval between the collection of samples and the supply of the vaccine, or else its administration by the practice that produced it, is only 14 days, and sometimes even considerably less. Within such a short space of time it is, at best, possible to isolate and multiply the pathogen, but not to conduct tests (e.g. to ensure that the pathogen in question has been safely inactivated by doing tests for sterility, residual toxicity {in the case of toxoid vaccines} or for residues of inactivation agents or preservatives).

Companies which perform such tests as part of their duty of care, and to satisfy certain minimum standards in relation to the manufacture and testing of herd-specific vaccines, are discriminated against as a result of the additional costs and the additional delays of several weeks before their vaccines are released on the market.

Adjustment to European Legislation

In summary IFAH-Europe believes that a series of changes in the EU legislation are required to harmonise and standardise rules for autogenous vaccines, especially with regard to the authorisation of veterinary autogenous vaccines, their production and control, labelling, batch-testing, use and the definition of herd-size. Autogenous vaccines are necessary for a herd- specific problem in a geographically "very limited" region, if no commercial vaccine is available. However, from the field it is known that problems of availability of licensed vaccines are occurring on a much wider scale, especially in the poultry sector, concerning more than one specific flock. The issue of vaccines for minor use and minor species have been addressed at this meeting. It should be kept in mind that industry would not develop certain vaccines as the return on investment is not justified. IFAH-Europe recommends that the production and use of autogenous vaccines be better regulated and controlled, as these types of vaccines would continue to be needed to ensure animal health and welfare and consumer safety.

Dr. S. Zänker, IFAH-Europe, 1, rue Defacqz, B-1000 Brussels, Belgium.
E-mail: szanker@ifahsec.org

Jungbäck C (ed): Consideration of Alternative Licensing Procedures for Vaccines for Minor Species, Minor Indications and Autogenous/Autologous Products.
Dev Biol. Basel, Karger, 2004, vol 117, p 31.

SESSION I (Part 2)

Autogenous/Autologous Vaccines

Identification of Suitable and Needed Antigens and Criteria for Quality of Production and Control

Moderator: *R. Hill* (CVB, USDA, APHIS)

Jungbäck C (ed): Consideration of Alternative Licensing Procedures for Vaccines for Minor Species, Minor Indications and Autogenous/Autologous Products.
Dev Biol. Basel, Karger, 2004, vol 117, pp 33-41.

Autologous Biologicals – Science/Regulations

M.L. Chapek, K.K. Brown, B.C. Lin

MVP Laboratories, Inc., Ralston, NE, USA

Reasons for Increased Interest in Autologous/Targeted Biologicals

There has been increased interest in Targeted Biologicals in the United States for several reasons. First, new technology is available to facilitate science-based isolate selection and manufacture. The science of Autologous/Targeted Biologicals will be discussed later in this presentation. A second reason for the increased interest in Targeted Biologicals is the fact that the livestock production methods have changed to favour herd/flock specific products controlled by a veterinarian. There have been changes in management methods such as segregated early weaning in swine, accelerated feeding and early weaning of dairy calves, and forced moulting in poultry. Herds and flocks have increased in stocking density and size. These factors stress animals and may facilitate mutation, strain variation and increased virulence of pathogens. Under these conditions, Traditional Biologicals may not be relevant to current field isolates. Many veterinarians favour vaccinating only for pathogens isolated from a herd/flock. A third reason for the increased interest in these products is that the licensing procedure for Targeted Biologicals is responsive to the needs of livestock producers. The process is abbreviated, requiring much less time and money. This allows for a more rapid response to emerging pathogens, strain variations and mutations, while facilitating the development of monovalent and multivalent products for limited markets or those for minor species.

Government Regulations

The licensing procedure for Targeted Biologicals does not allow the sale of live attenuated or recombinant products because these would require more extensive safety testing. Government regulations are the same for Traditional and Targeted Biologicals regarding licensing of facilities, approval of personnel, product licence documentation and unannounced USDA inspections. They are also the same for testing primary cells and cell lines [1]. Cell line testing regulations include karyology, purity, adventitious agents (confirmed by government), mycoplasma and animal origin ingredient testing. Regulations relating to documentation of Master Seed differ in some aspects. The isolation and passage history is necessary for both product types, as is identification except, in the interest of a timely response to the veterinarian/producer, for the first serial of Targeted Biologicals from a given isolate. Extensive purity testing is performed on Master Seeds of Traditional Biologicals, but not the seeds of Targeted Biologicals. The Master Seeds for the latter are animal isolates. Typically, there are minimal in vitro passages made from the isolate, helping to assure retention of herd-relevant antigens. Often the seeds of Traditional Products are passaged numerous times to obtain adequate stocks of Master and Working Seeds to last possibly for decades. To use an isolate beyond 15 months but no more than 24 months, manufacturers of Targeted Biologicals are required to document efficacy and lack of adverse reactions in the field, provide an assessment of herd health status, and document a veterinarian/client/patient relationship. Manufacturers of Traditional Biologicals are not required to provide proof of any of the above and may continue the use of a particular isolate in a herd or flock indefinitely.

Manufacturers of Traditional Products predict field performance by conducting a host animal immunogenicity test, which may use an artificial challenge method with an isolate that is not necessarily characteristic of current field pathogens. The results may not reflect a product's performance under actual field conditions. They are also required to perform a host animal safety study before licensing. Manufacturers of Targeted Biologicals, on the other hand, anticipate field performance by incorporating isolates that are relevant to the disease problems in a herd or flock and by minimizing in vitro passages.

Government regulations for production documentation are the same for both product types regarding Outlines of Production, Special Outlines, extraneous agent testing of animal origin ingredients, batch records and product labelling.

Quality Control regulations that are the same for Traditional and Targeted Biologicals are formaldehyde determination, testing of ingredients for mycoplasma contamination, government retention samples, government release of serials, sterility and safety testing. However, the first serial of a Targeted Biological made with a given isolate may be released after three days of testing for sterility and safety, provided the tests are satisfactory at that time. The tests are continued and serials must be recalled if a problem develops. Regulations relating to potency testing differ in that a serial release potency test is required for Traditional Biologicals, while Targeted Biologicals must contain isolates from sick or dead animals, giving them herd/flock relevance.

Duration of immunity studies may be required for new entities and special cases of Traditional, but not Targeted products. Retrospective stability testing is required for Traditional Biologicals because they are manufactured months to years before use, whereas Targeted Biologicals are made to order and typically are to be used quickly.

Selection of Suitable Isolates

New molecular technologies such as PCR and DNA sequencing have become increasingly important methods for diagnostic laboratories and manufacturers of

Targeted Biologicals. These techniques provide a rapid means to identify, characterize and select the most suitable isolates for use in such products. The manufacture of Targeted Biologicals requires a close collaboration between a state-of-the-art diagnostic laboratory and the herd/flock veterinarian. The veterinarian sends appropriate tissues and/or body fluids from diseased animals to the diagnostic laboratory that identifies and characterizes potential pathogens. The laboratory findings are discussed and a determination is made regarding which isolates are most suitable to address the herd/flock health problems.

Figures 1 to 4 demonstrate the importance of molecular methods for use in selecting suitable isolates for incorporation into Targeted Biologicals [2]. Figure 1 shows the PCR amplification pattern of the R1 repeat region of the p97 adhesin gene from some field isolates of *Mycoplasma hyopneumoniae* received by MVP Laboratories over a period of a year as compared with the same region from DNA extracted from seven Traditional *M. hyopneumoniae* products. The sizes of the p97 R1 repeat gene are ≥ 300 bp. In contrast, the size of the same gene region from the field isolates is < 280 bp. This variation may seem trivial. However, Hsu and Minion have reported that the cilium binding site of *M. hyopneumoniae* is located in this p97 gene sequence [3]. More specifically, Minion et al published that only three repeat units (15 amino acids) are needed for defining the p97 binding epitope [4]. Therefore, it can be postulated that any change in the R1 repeat region of this gene may prevent the binding of antibodies that are specific for the original epitope. These seemingly small variations in the p97 gene of the field isolates, as compared with that region of the isolates found in the Traditional Biologicals, may explain the lack of protection often observed with such products. Targeted Biologicals would include isolates containing the relevant p97 gene sequence. Figure 2 demonstrates the use of PCR to determine the species of Mycoplasma isolated from two separate cases. In a rapid test that requires only a couple of hours, it can be determined that

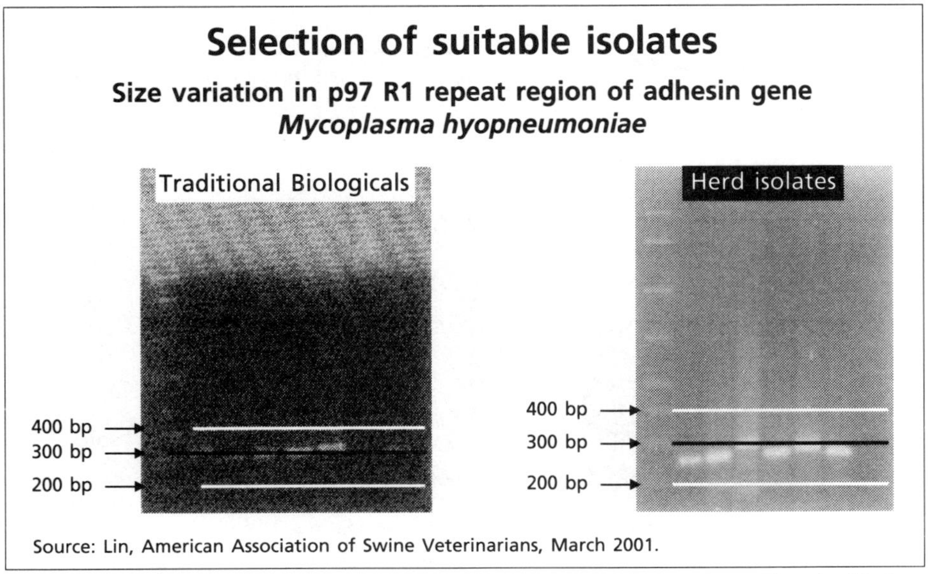

Fig. 1: Comparison of the R1 repeat region of p97 gene of *Mycoplasma hyopneumoniae* from herd isolates with strains from Traditional Biologicals.

Selection of suitable isolates

Use of PCR for identification of mycoplasma genus and species

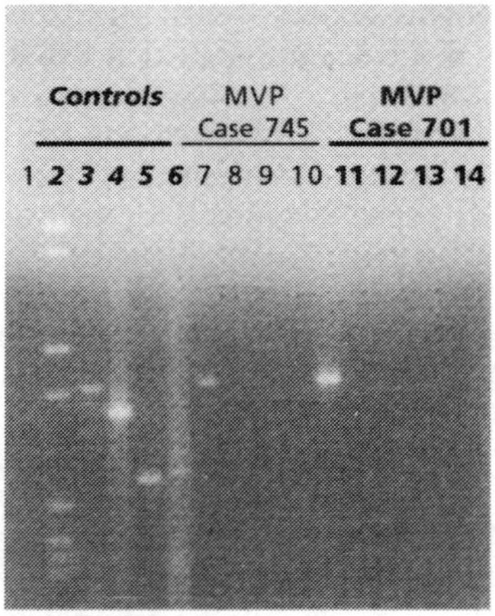

1. Blank
2. ***DNA ladder***
3. ***M. hyopneumoniae***
4. ***M. hyorhinis***
5. ***M. hyosynoviae***
6. ***M. flocculare***
7. Unknow isolate MVP case 745
8. Unknow isolate MVP case 745
9. Unknow isolate MVP case 745
10. Unknow isolate MVP case 745
11. **Unknow isolate MVP case 701**
12. **Unknow isolate MVP case 701**
13. **Unknow isolate MVP case 701**
14. **Unknow isolate MVP case 701**

Source: MVP Laboratories, Inc.

Fig. 2: Use of PCR for identification of the genus and species of *Mycoplasma hyopneumoniae* isolates.

Selection of suitable isolates

PCR characterization of *Haemophilus parasuis*

RFLP genotype

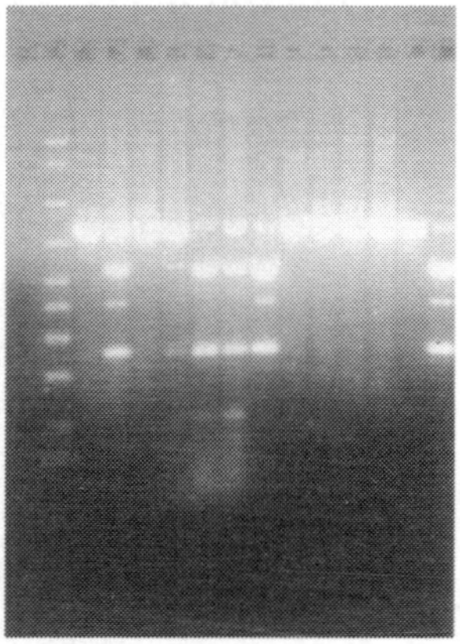

Lane	Serotype	RFLP
3	*NT*	*1A*
4	13	3A
5	4	1A
6	4	1B
7	4	2A
8	4	3A
9	4	2B
10	*NT*	*1A*
11	2	1A
12	4	1A
13	*NT*	*1A*
14	4	1A
15	4	1B

NT = Nontypeable

Source: Lin, American Association of Swine Veterinarians, March 2003.

Fig. 3: Use of PCR to characterize *Haemophilus parasuis* isolates to differentiate nontypeables and isolates within serotypes.

the isolates from cases 745 and 701 are *M. hyopneumoniae* [2]. Figure 3 shows the added value of PCR when evaluating isolates of *Haemophilus parasuis* [5]. Isolates of this organism are normally identified by serotyping. Fifteen serotypes are known. However, there are numerous isolates obtained that are non-typable (NT). By using PCR genotyping, the non-typable isolates can be differentiated. Additionally, differentiation within a single serotype can be made (as represented by serotype 4 in the slide). Figure 4 represents the importance of using molecular techniques to select a suitable isolate for a Targeted Biological containing *Clostridium difficile*. Two different isolates were obtained from a single case. Both isolates were identified as *C. difficile* by normal biochemical identification procedures. However, after PCR analysis, it was determined that isolate #1 contained the genes for both the A and B toxin while isolate #2 contained genes for neither toxin. Isolate 1 was chosen for incorporation into the Targeted Biological. If isolate 2 had been chosen for the product, the critical protective toxoid could not have been prepared and the herd probably would not have been protected.

Selection of suitable isolates

MVP case 10219

Clostridium difficile toxin gene analysis

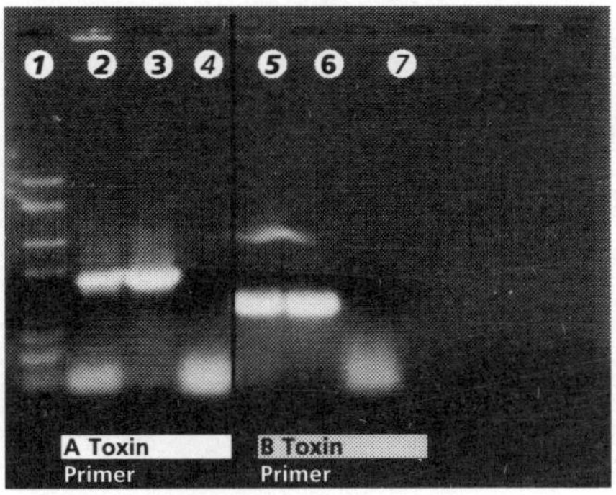

Lane 1	***DNA ladder***
Lanes 2 and 5	***Know strain containing both A and both B toxin genes***
Lanes 3 and 6	**Isolate 1 Positive for A and B toxins**
Lanes 4 and 7	*Isolate 2 Negative for A and B toxins*

Isolate 1 was used for manufacture of Targeted Biological

Source: MVP Laboratories, Inc.

Fig. 4: Use of PCR to select the correct isolate from two *Clostridium difficile* organisms obtained from the same tissue sample.

Quality and Consistency of Production

After the selection of suitable isolates, the process of production is begun. This includes customizing the formulation to the herd of origin by further discussing the herd problems with the veterinarian to determine the combinations, proportions, dose and vial size. Adjuvant selection is based on the diseases requiring protection and is critical because Targeted Biologicals are inactivated. If protection is antibody-dependent, an adjuvant such as Emulsigen® may be used. If protection is

T-cell dependent, an adjuvant incorporating a T-cell stimulating component may be selected (Polygen™ or Carbigen™). After selection of the adjuvant system to use, there is a discussion and decision on the most appropriate vaccination schedule, which is included on the product label.

Although there may not be specific requirements for characterization of growth, harvest, inactivation and adjuvants for various pathogens, any manufacturer interested in producing quality products that will perform well in the field will conduct such studies. Product quality is, at least in part, a reflection of the manufacturer's integrity. Figures 5 to 9 demonstrate the types of evaluations that MVP and other ethical manufacturers conduct, on a periodical basis, in order to manufacture immunogenic biologicals consistently. Figure 5 illustrates that it is important to evaluate media ingredients for their growth-promoting characteristics. In the case of yeast extract, MVP has determined that, in most cases, better yields of organisms can be obtained with fresh yeast extract produced in-house rather than powdered yeast extract purchased from a third party. Figure 6 shows a growth curve for *Streptococcus suis,* used to establish the optimum harvest time. This helps to ensure that there is adequate antigenic mass for each isolate. Figures 7 and 8 indicate an additional method conducted to select the optimum harvest time for antigen production, as well as the optimum inactivation method. These slides relate to the retention of antigens known to be immunogenic for *Mycoplasma bovis*. It is noted in Figure 7 that the important antigens decrease slightly after 24 hours of growth, probably due to a protease, so the harvest time for this organism is

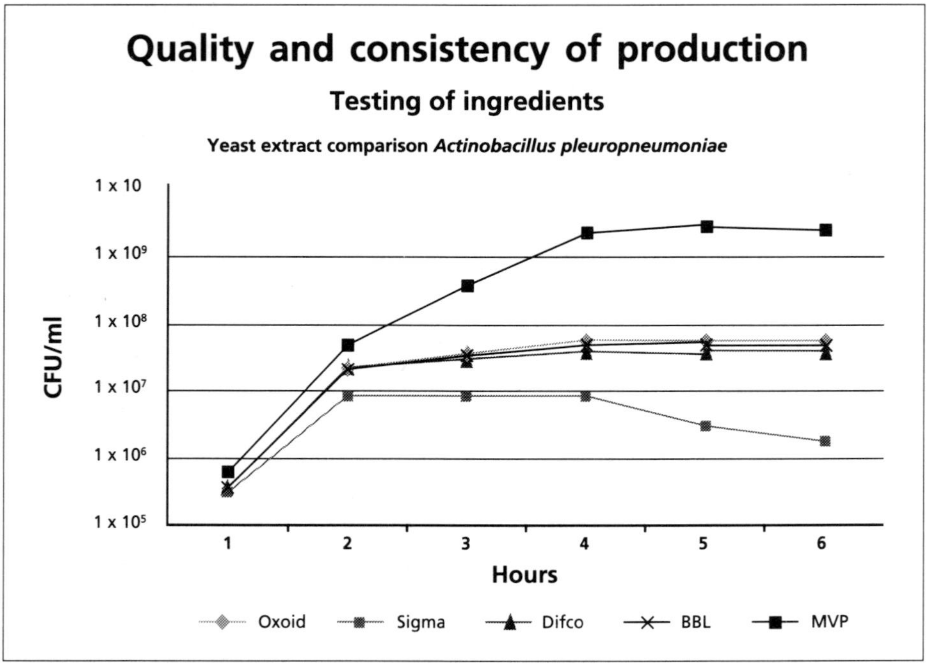

Fig. 5: Testing of ingredients such as yeast extract is important to obtain the highest antigenic mass for the product.

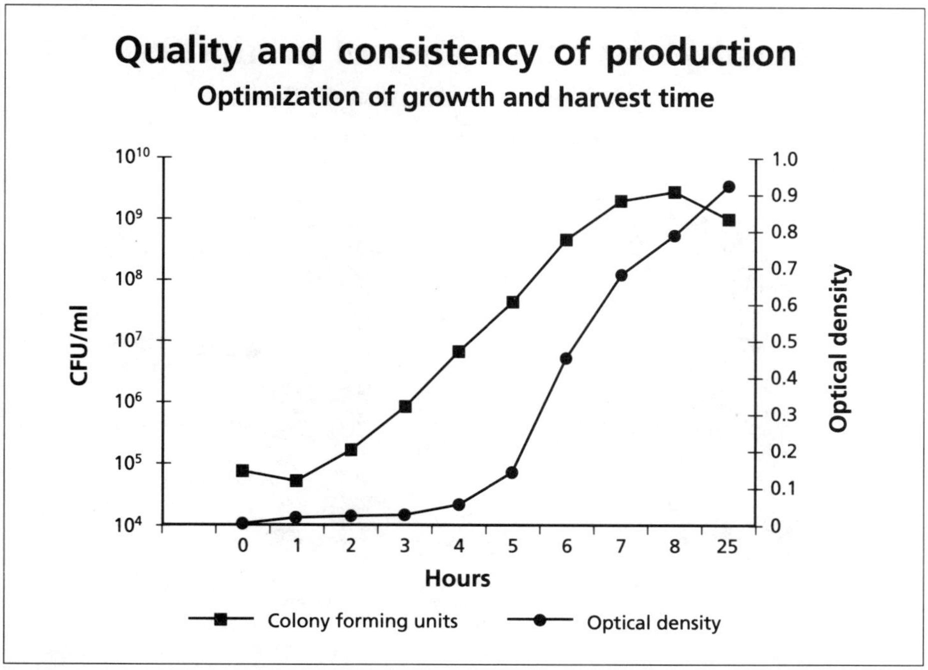

Fig. 6: Optimization of growth and harvest time base on optical density and colony forming units for *Streptococcus suis.*

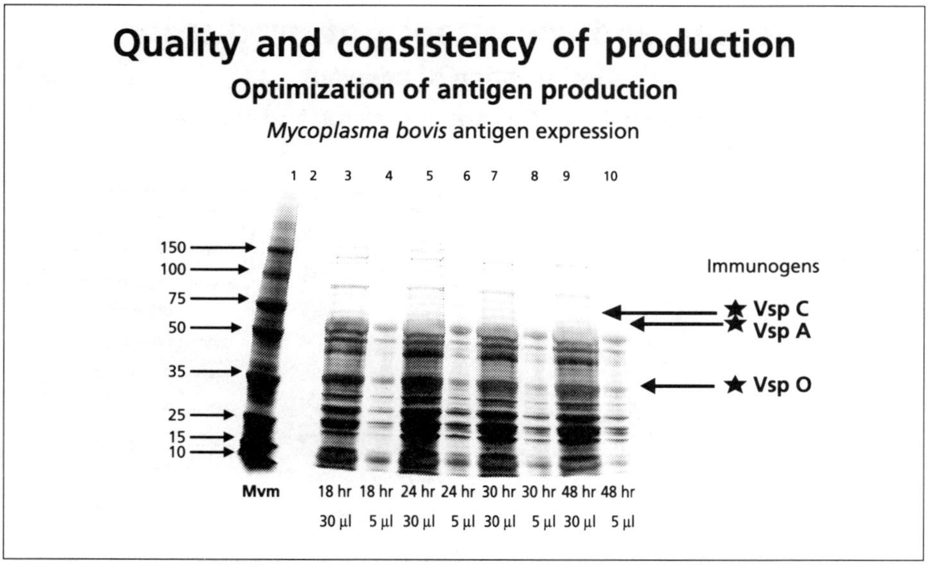

Fig. 7: Optimization of antigen production to ensure the presence of immunogens.

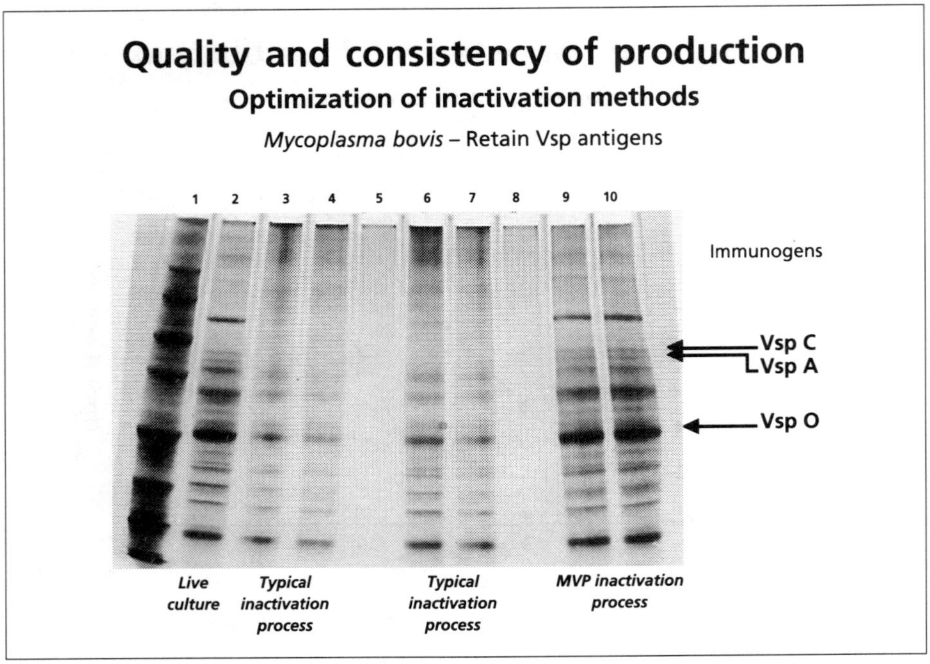

Fig. 8: Optimization of inactivating agent so as to retain important antigens.

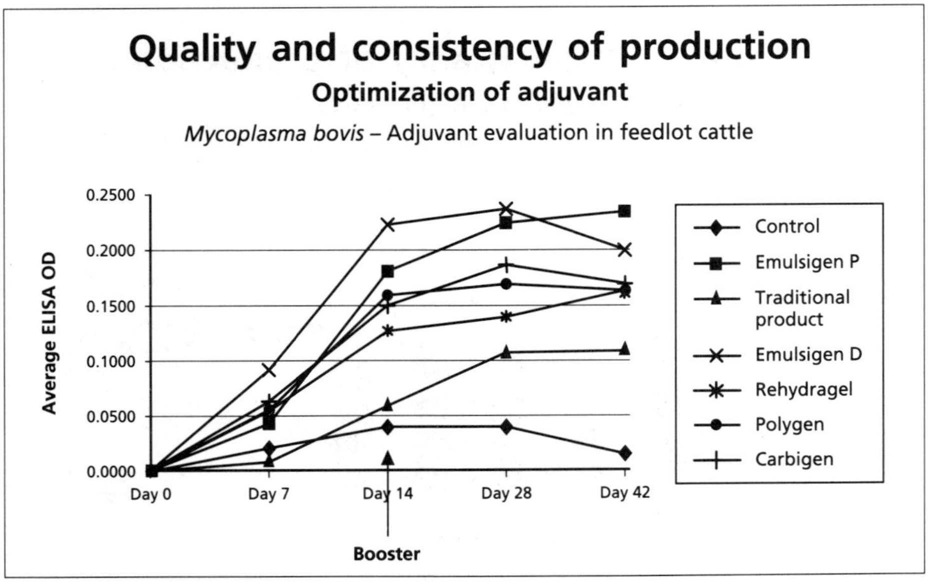

Fig. 9: Optimization of adjuvant to antigen is critical in ensuring performance of product.

optimally 18 hours. From Figure 8 it is apparent that certain inactivating agents totally destroy the important antigens. Without harvest time determination and use of the correct inactivating agent, the Targeted Biological would probably not protect. Figure 9 demonstrates the importance of evaluating adjuvants and their effectiveness with each antigen. Such studies are not required for either Traditional or Targeted Biologicals. Targeted Biologicals have the advantage of using the best adjuvant for the product if the manufacturer has multiple adjuvants approved.

Advantages of Targeted Biologicals

There are numerous advantages of Targeted Biologicals over Traditional Biologicals. These include: (i) providing rapid response to new pathogens and relevant mutations; (ii) inclusion of isolates in the product that are specific for the herd pathogens; (iii) allowing selection of adjuvants most appropriate for the pathogen; (iv) providing products for limited markets; (v) requiring collaboration with a licensed veterinarian; and (vi) addressing customer demand for selection of antigens and control of prices.

Conclusion

The reality is that there is increased interest from veterinarians and livestock producers in Targeted Biologicals in the U.S. This increased interest is led by the development of new molecular technologies that facilitate science-based selection of isolates and manufacture of Targeted Biologicals. Finally, it takes both government regulators and manufacturer integrity to ensure that quality products are available to the veterinarians and producers, whether these products are Traditional or Targeted Biologicals.

References

1 Code of Federal Regulations, Title 9, Government Printing Office, Washington, DC, 2003.

2 Lin BC: Intraspecies differentiation of *Mycoplasma hyopneumoniae* field strains isolated in the United States. Proceedings of the 31st Annual Meeting of American Association of Swine Veterinarians, Indianapolis, IN, 2001, pp 225-235.

3 Hsu T, Minion FC: Identification of the Cilium Binding Epitope of the *Mycoplasma hyopneumoniae* p97 Adhesin. Infect Immun 1998; 66: 4762-4766.

4 Minion FC, Adams C, Hsu T: R1 Region of p97 Mediates Adherence of *Mycoplasma hyopneumoniae* to Swine Cilia. Infect Immun 2000; 68: 3056-3060.

5 Lin BC: Identification and differentiation of *Haemophilus parasuis* sero-nontypeable strains using a species-specific PCR and the digestion of PCR products with HindIII endonuclease. Proceedings of the 33rd Annual Meeting of American Association of Swine Veterinarians, Orlando, FL, 2003, pp 299-301.

Mrs. M.-L. Chapek, MVP Laboratories, Inc., 5404 Miller Ave., Ralston, NE 68127, USA.
E-mail: marylou@mvplabs.com

Jungbäck C (ed): Consideration of Alternative Licensing Procedures for Vaccines for Minor Species, Minor Indications and Autogenous/Autologous Products.
Dev Biol. Basel, Karger, 2004, vol 117, pp 43-47.

Autogenous Vaccines: Determining Product Need and Antigen Selection, Production and Testing Considerations

H.A. Draayer

Pfizer Animal Health, Richland, MI, USA

Abstract: It is estimated that in the 12-month period from May 1999-April 2000 approximately \$16.06 million in swine autogenous vaccines were sold in the United States. Swine influenza and PRRS vaccines accounted for over one-half of these sales. Usage patterns suggest USDA regulation covering the production and use of autogenous vaccines may be violated. A proposal for product use and selection criteria that may minimize the potential for abuse of autogenous regulations is described. Using a decision tree, the analysis considers issues such as availability of registered products, recognized strain variations and the current state of vaccine technology. Proposed testing and production scenarios are described that include food safety considerations, yet allow for the rapid production and testing required for autogenous products.

INTRODUCTION

In a survey commissioned by Pfizer Animal Health, C.F. Grass Consulting estimated that during the 12-month period for May 1999 — April 2000, autogenous vaccines sales for the United States swine market, at the manufacturer level were approximately \$16.6 million. Leading these sales were Swine Flu product accounting for 35% of sales, PRRS 21%, *Step/A. suis* 15%, *H. parasius* 13%, *Mycoplasma* 10%. The remaining 6% consisted of products such as APP, *Cl. Perfringens* type A, *E. coli* F18 etc. Expectations obtained during this survey were that the rate of autogenous sales would grow at double the rate of commercial vaccines. Three US producers accounted for more that 96% of these swine autogenous sales: Newport Labs (54%), Imm Tech Biological (26%) and MPV (16.8%).

In this survey, the most commonly sited positive aspects for autogenous vaccine use were: (i) these vaccines use a customized approach to vaccination, focusing on the individual herd and diseases; (ii) vaccines are available at a lower cost and can be used by the veterinarian as a revenue builder (iii) in certain cases, commercial vaccines are perceived as ineffective, and (iv) it was easier to obtain the desired combination vaccines from the autogenous producers.

On the negative side, veterinarians felt that: (i) these vaccines were not always safe or effective; (ii) the antigen dose in the vaccine was often based on assumptions; (iii) the vaccines take too long to obtain from the producers; (iv) the vaccine strains must be re-isolated on a yearly basis; (v) there was not enough governmental oversight and control, and (vi) these vaccines underwent minimal testing before sale.

In the United States, autogenous vaccines are regulated by the United States Department of Agriculture, Center for Veterinary Biologics. In a tiered system of registration requirements, autogenous vaccines are the least regulated. Conditionally licensed vaccines follow autogenous vaccines and finally fully licensed products. This tiered system is designed to meet market and emerging disease situations. The basic tenets of USDA's autogenous regulations include the following:

(i) autogenous vaccines must be inactivated and non-toxic;

(ii) autogenous vaccines must be used by the veterinarian, or under veterinarian client-patient relationship;

(iii) autogenous vaccines must be isolated from the herd of origin, and in most cases limited to that herd (possible adjacent herd exemptions are available);

(iv) autogenous vaccines can contain multiple organisms;

(v) organisms used for autogenous vaccine production cannot be used for more than 15 months from the date of the first isolation or 12 months from the date of harvest. These times can be extended if specific requirements are met;

(vi) autogenous vaccines must be tested for purity and lab animal safety;

(vii) autogenous vaccines must be released by USDA's Center for Veterinary Biologics before shipping;

(viii) autogenous vaccines will have 18-month dating.

Product Need, Antigen Selection Considerations

The basic concept of autogenous vaccines is to make products available to veterinarians and producers in cases where conventional vaccines are proving ineffective, or are not available. Regulations governing autogenous vaccines should be based on this basic concept. To address this need, autogenous regulations should be designed to ask the following questions before authorizing the use of these products:

(i) are there registered (licensed) veterinary biologicals available to address the disease need? Have the products been used in the herd in question, and have they been shown to be ineffective? Are there underlying management issues that may contribute to the perceived lack of efficacy (i.e. maternal antibody interference)?

(ii) if there are no registered products available, is there a scientific basis for this lack of licensed products? Is the lack of products based on recent strain drifts, emerging diseases or limited market (i.e. minor species)?

(iii) is the disease caused by an agent with multiple serotypes or documented antigenic drift?

(iv) do herd size, integration and/or management practices have an impact on the proper use of the vaccines?

Figure 1 represents a proposed decision tree that can be used to help evaluated potential autogenous vaccine usage, based on the above considerations.

As indicated previously, USDA regulations were developed to address disease issues in the isolation herd. Exemptions were also developed to define adjacent herds, and use of the vaccines in these herds. With the increase in integration in the United States and other markets, originally in the poultry industry, but also in swine and cattle, this definition may need to be reconsidered. When developing new autogenous vaccine regulations, the definition of the herd should include all premises operated by an integrated operation where personnel and animals are shared.

Product Testing Considerations

A key factor required for the use of autogenous vaccines is to minimize the interval between isolation and use of the vaccine. By its nature, this premise entails compromises in the testing of vaccine serials before release. However, in

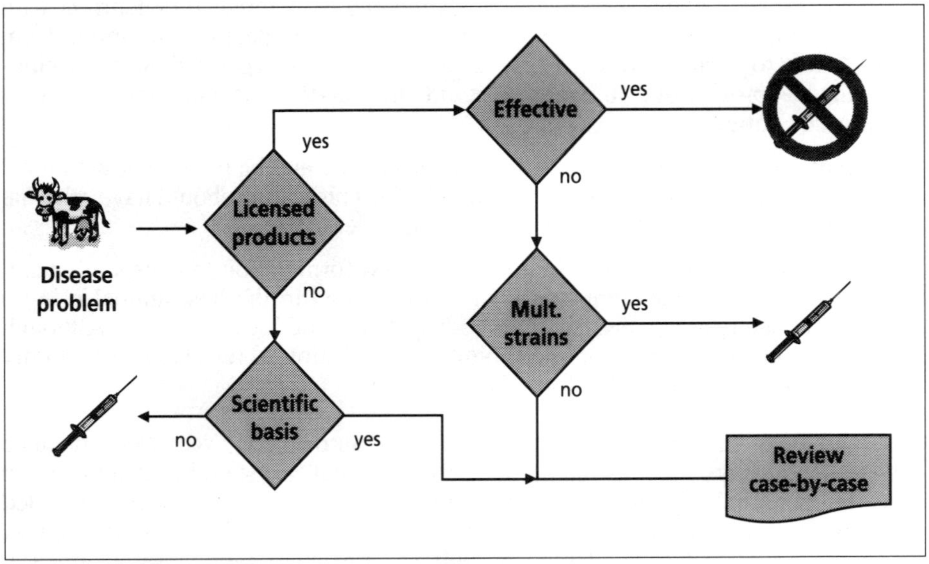

Fig. 1: Decision tree for autogenous vaccine use justification.

developing new legislation, two factors should not be compromised: (i) potential contamination of vaccines with extraneous agents, including TSE's and reportable diseases (e.g. BHV-1 in certain areas of the EU); (ii) factors that have an impact on the safety of the food supply.

To minimize the potential risks, the following testing requirements are proposed, in addition to those currently in place in the United States. Some tests, as indicated, can be conducted concurrently with product release, as long as traceability and recall provisions are in place.

1. All raw materials used in the production of autogenous vaccines, in particular those of biological origin, should be held to the same testing standards, and production standards as those used for licensed vaccines. This includes testing for extraneous contamination, inactivation and inactivation validation where appropriate. All requirements designed to limit the risk of TSE should be incorporated, including documentation of the source. This testing/documentation can all be done in advance and should have no impact on the timing from isolation to serial release.
2. Cell lines used for the production of viral seeds should undergo full testing (as is currently required by the USDA for autogenous vaccines). Again, this testing/documentation can all be done in advance and should have no impact on the timing from isolation to serial release.
3. Viral isolates should be subject to at least limited extraneous testing. In cases where rapid test procedures are not available (i.e. PCR) this testing can be completed concurrent to serial release as along as recall provisions are in place, in case positive results are obtained.
4. As under the USDA system, isolates should be identified to, at a minimum, the genus level before use. In addition, testing should be completed where possible to species, strain and serotype. This testing can be completed concurrent with first serial release, and should have no or minimal impact on the timing from isolation to serial release. These data could be incorporated in a vaccino-vigilance programme to monitor strain drift and/or the emergence of new disease entities
5. Serials should be tested for residual formaldehyde and be compliant with local maximum formaldehyde levels before release. This testing should have minimal impact on the timing from isolation to serial release.
6. To help assure food safety, "first use" of a new formulation (e.g. new adjuvant, major change in excipients etc.), should be tested in the host animal using a standard safety assay observing for both systemic and local reactions. Although this will have an impact on the timing from isolation to release, this will only occur once for each unique formulation.

To reduce the potential for abuse with autogenous vaccines adequate governmental supervision is required. The United States system has demonstrated that the potential for abuse exists in the use of original isolates, extended distribution, and extend use of an isolate. To minimize this potential abuse, resources need to be available to address use justification, serial release, distribution issues and also have the power to enforce compliance.

Conclusions

Autogenous vaccines provide an additional tool for both veterinarians and the veterinary biologicals industry. By rapidly bring vaccines to select herds; these vaccines can fill a void left by the current stringent requirements to bring a new isolate through the registration process. With proper reporting these products can serve as an early warning system for strain variations and emerging diseases. In addition data generated by specific vaccines could supply a manufacture with a faster course to a fully licensed veterinary biological.

Reference

1 Grass CF: Autogenous Vaccine Market Analysis. A proprietary consulting Project, G.F. Grass Consulting, May 2000.

Dr. H.A. Draayer, Pfizer Animal Health, 0225-190-43, 5300 N. 28th St., Richland, MI 49083, USA.
E-mail: Hans_Draayer@groton.pfizer.com

Jungbäck C (ed): Consideration of Alternative Licensing Procedures for Vaccines for Minor Species, Minor Indications and Autogenous/Autologous Products.
Dev Biol. Basel, Karger, 2004, vol 117, pp 49-53.

The Manufacture of Autogenous Vaccines in France

C. Miras

Agence Française de Sécurité Sanitaire des Aliments, Agence Nationale du Médicament Vétérinaire, Fougères, France

The presentation consists of an introduction of the French experience concerning the control of autogenous vaccines: the current and future reflection on the status of these products and the implementation of a legislation intended to define legal bounds for the manufacture and the distribution of these particular medicinal products.

In France, autogenous vaccines are not allowed in the human field but can be used in the veterinary field as an answer to specific pathological cases. These products are out of the scope of the European regulations in force relating to veterinary medicinal products (Directive 2001/82/CEE). Currently, French legislation regarding specifically autogenous vaccines comprises only a few points: (i) the current situation of the legislation existing on autogenous vaccines in France; (ii) a comment on the current field situation and (iii) a focus on some aspects of the specificity of these products and (iv) on ways of implementing some of the regulatory requirements.

The definition of these products is as follows: autogenous vaccines are veterinary medicinal products prepared from pathogens from an animal or animals from the same holding, inactivated and used for the active immunisation of an animal or animals from the same holding. The second point of the legislation mentions the following requirement: the manufacture of autogenous vaccines and veterinary use must be performed by a person holding an authorisation granted by the AFSSA-ANMV.

Some other legal requirements, national or European, apply to autogenous vaccines which are not specific to these products: with all medicinal products, autogenous vaccines should conform with the legal requirements concerning MRL, TSE, and the absence of glycol ethers in the composition. All legislation in force which may be applicable to autogenous products must be respected and particularly regulation concerning prophylaxis.

The current field situation such as perceived by our authority is as follows: the need for autogenous vaccines in the veterinary field.

Use of autogenous vaccines can be conceivable to address particular situations, such as a totally new infectious disease involving a new pathogen. To fight against the spread of a new infection, an autogenous vaccine may be considered as a first solution before use of a traditional vaccine; given that development of a new vaccine would take a long time and that according to the epidemiological situation of this disease (species, spread of infection,...) production of a conventional vaccine may not appear as an interesting development for vaccine manufacturers. In the absence of an authorised vaccine: for minor species or minor indications, few authorised vaccines are available and use of autogenous vaccines may be a response for the control of some infectious disease not covered by authorised products.

Considering these particular cases, it should be stressed that autogenous vaccines should not be in competition with medicinal products with marketing authorisation. Autogenous vaccines should be considered as alternative medicine to be used in particular justified circumstances and submitted to the European regulation concerning the "cascade principle (autogenous vaccines assimilated to extemporaneous preparations).

To take stock of the situation in the AFSSA-ANMV and of the situation in the field: currently, 11 persons have the legal authorisation to produce autogenous vaccines. These authorisations were delivered between 1982 and 2003 (one recent authorisation). Earlier authorisations have not been updated since 1986. No follow-up of the authorised persons nor their activities has been performed since the granting of these authorisations.

Production and distribution of autogenous vaccines appear as a recrudescent activity with production of many millions of doses. Apart from some autogenous vaccines consisting of crushed "warts" (papillomas), all autogenous vaccines are inactivated bacterial vaccines intended principally for food species (poultry, porcine, fish).

Inspections organised recently by the AFSSA-ANMV in many laboratories manufacturing antugenous vaccines reveal that manufacturing conditions and controls performed by the different laboratories were very heterogeneous and in the majority of cases did not conform with European Pharmacopeia requirements for regional vaccines (sterility test, safety test....).

In the analysis of the current situation, the necessity for setting up a national legislation should be stressed which will aim to:

(i) revise the current authorisations which have never been actualised;

(ii) define or redefine the notion of autogenous vaccines itself: criteria for use, conditions of use, prescription, manufacture and delivery in field situation;

(iii) define more precisely the conditions of granting the authorisation to manufacture autogenous vaccines;

(iv) define legal requirements to assess a minimal level of quality for these products, through the implementation of Good Manufacturing Practices for autogenous vaccines and the definition of minimal controls for these products.

There are some specific considerations regarding autogenous vaccines which need some reflection. The manufacture and distribution of conventional vaccines are controlled by national authorities through granting of a marketing authorisation. This MA results from the assessment of a complete file which allows the national authority to assess a level of quality, safety and efficacy for the product which appears for the user in the SPC. For autogenous vaccines, it is impossible to assess quality, safety and efficacy in the same way. Manufacture of these products is performed following prescription: all products contain specific infectious agents; qualitative and quantitative composition of these products is poorly standardized. It should be considered that the laboratory which manufactures these products is responsible for the quality of production, safety and efficacy of its products. Through requirements and inspections, the national authority can only assess a minimal level of quality for the production of autogenous vaccines, assessing an obligation of means of production, but not an obligation of the results.

The definition of autogenous vaccines mentions that the active ingredient of an autogenous vaccine is obtained from pathogens from an animal or animals from the same holding and must be used for the active immunisation of this animal or animals from the same holding (production site). It should be underlined that this current definition appears poorly adapted to the field situation considering the current structure of holdings. We can ask ourselves how field situations will be managed considering the current practices. In practice, for many food animals, production such as poultry (layers, breeders) pigs (fattening, nursery) or fish, animals are moved from one specific holding site to another which is geographically and sometimes administratively different, according to category. It may be that veterinarians consider the need to vaccinate the upstream holding site, to protect the downstream holding site where the infectious agent has been isolated, and where animals will be moved to ensure the immunity of these animals before the introduction in the contaminated site. The current definition of autogenous vaccine does not allow this practice. Revision of the current definition of autogenous vaccines to include the concept of epidemiological unit seems necessary and needs further reflection.

It should be underlined that the concept of epidemiological unit has not been retained by the Europe Commission (See Directive 2001/82/CEE, Titre II, article 3, chapter 2).

Project of Legislation in France

The authorisation will be granted to a qualified person in collaboration with the production site. The following points have been retained to define the nature of the authorisation: (i) the authorised person will be responsible for the quality/safety/efficacy of the autogenous vaccines produced and for compliance of the release productions with legislation in force; (ii) autogenous vaccines should be delivered to the veterinarian who has isolated the infectious agent and ordered the prescription. This person is responsible for the administration of the products in the field. Granting of the authorisation would be based on the assessment of a request: the request should mention the name of the applicant, site of production, a list of antigens/adjuvants intended to be used for the production and should contain a technical dossier. The assessment performed by the authority is different from the assessment of a Marketing authorisation dossier and is more similar to the assessment of manufacturers' authorisation. The following points have been retained to define the nature of the assessment: (i) the assessment would be based on examination of the request (qualification of the applicant) and particularly the examination of the list of antigens/adjuvants intended to be used for the manufacture of autogenous vaccines; (ii) the applicant should confirm this compliance with regulation concerning (TSE, MRL and so on).

Granting of the authorisation will be principally based on the results of the inspection of the proposed manufacturing site. The technical dossier provided by the applicant should describe the process from sampling of the infectious agent and its identification and purification to the delivery of the autogenous vaccine to the veterinarian who ordered the prescription.

All the traceability system should be detailed: inspection which will check the conformity of the manufacturing process with the process described in the technical dossier and with the legal requirements in force; Good Manufacturing Practices for production of autogenous vaccines should be defined. They should be similar to the current GMP with some alleviations of requirements defined in relation with the specificity of these products. Requirements concerning the upstream steps (prescription, sampling, and transportation of samples) as well as downstream steps (transportation and delivery) should also be adequately specified and will be similar to requirements existing for veterinary medicinal products (prescription similar to the prescription of an extemporaneous preparation,..) .

The following point should be stressed: the authorisation will integrate a list of antigens and adjuvants which can be used for the production of autogenous vaccines. This list will specify antigens that may be used for production in connection with target species and disease; it will be assessed by the national authority which will check the conformity of the proposed list with legislation (absence of active ingredient already included in an authorised immunological product, absence of prophylaxis regulation for the active ingredients in question....). This would prevent manufacturers from producing and releasing autogenous vaccines if a vaccine with an MA already exists for the same species/same indications. Specific needs for autogenous vaccines even in the presence of authorised products should then be justified by the applicant (supportive veterinarians data). The authorisation would be delivered for five days after a maximum assessment of 120 days. This authorisation should be subject to renewal every five years.

Each change should be declared by the manufacturer and will be treated as a variation and be assessed by the AFSSA-ANMV (30 days + eventually 120 days according to the nature of change and need of inspections). This change can concern addition of an active ingredient/adjuvant. Each variation that may change the content of the request or the content of the technical dossier has to be declared and examined by the authority. In the case of the granting of a new Marketing Authorisation for a new vaccine that contains an infectious agent usually included in the qualitative composition of autogenous vaccines, authorisations may be revised. The list of authorised antigens to be used and annexed to the authorisation may be officially activated by the administrative powers.

As with all veterinary products, autogenous vaccines may be followed in the field through the pharmaco-vigilance system. All adverse reactions as well as lack of efficacy have to be declared to the AFSSA-ANMV through the current pharmaco-vigilance system. Requests for renewal should contain all pharmaco-vigilance data obtained by the producer.

Importations of autogenous vaccines from other European countries may be possible. Veterinarians can send their prescription to manufacturers from other countries. Each request will be examined as individual importations from documents and dossiers such as described in the legislation regarding importations. In the absence of European regulations on autogenous vaccines, requirements in many countries are not necessarily harmonised and authorisation granted in a European country currently cannot be recognised as such by the French authority; specific assessment of a request should be effected by the French authority whatever the location of the manufacturing site, and treated as an importation request. However, it should be mentioned that importations of autogenous vaccines might meet difficulties with the circulation of biological samples across frontiers (such circulation cannot be managed by the AFSSA/ANMV).

Conclusion

It should be pointed out that this brief reflection is continuing; the project of regulation has been submitted to the European Community. So all points tackled represent the French national authority vision/perception of autogenous vaccines and may be revised after decisions/assessment by Europe and after some years of experience of such a legislation. Perhaps we can hope in a few years to have some European vision and regulation related to autogenous vaccines.

Dr. C. Miras, Agence Française de Sécurité Sanitaires des Aliments, Agence Nationale du Médicament Vétérinaire, La Haute Marche, B.P. 203 Javené, F-35302 Fougères, France.
E-mail: c.miras@anmv.afssa.fr

Jungbäck C (ed): Consideration of Alternative Licensing Procedures for Vaccines for Minor Species, Minor Indications and Autogenous/Autologous Products.
Dev Biol. Basel, Karger, 2004, vol 117, pp 55-60.

Current Concepts and Future Approaches to the Development of Autologous/Autogenous Vaccines for Veterinary Use

M. Tollis

Laboratorio di Medicina Veterinaria, Istituto Superiore di Sanità, Roma, Italy

Abstract: Current classification of autologous/autogenous (A/A) vaccines is commonly based on the concept of strain/antigen specificity associated with targeted treatment of a restricted number of animals. However, fulfilling these two conditions is not sufficient for immune-veterinary immune-biologicals to be excluded from the provisions of Directive 2001/82/EC. Indeed, non-inactivated A/A vaccines are not automatically considered out of the scope of the community code relating to veterinary medicinal products, in particular to immune-biologicals. As a major consequence of the "regulatory" exclusion from the requirements of EU rules, A/A vaccines can be usually manufactured and distributed without having obtained a marketing authorization by the competent authority of a Member State. Furthermore, strain specificity enables veterinarians to consider the use of these vaccines in quite a large variety of epidemiological circumstances where no "conventional" vaccines are yet available or are considered efficacious. In addition, in contrast to "conventional" vaccines, which are considered exclusively as a preventive tool against infectious diseases, A/A vaccines can also be used to treat "continuing" infections. Although the limited scientific value of these products and the poor investigations of the effector mechanisms involved are widely recognized, their use is still claimed in conditions where disorders in the immune system are suspected. Today, a more appropriate definition of A/A vaccines is one that takes into account their historical tradition and practical use, such as stable- or herd-specific vaccines, custom ("..ized") vaccines, therapeutic vaccines, pharmavaccines, vaccines used for biological therapy, etc. Although acknowledging the "regulatory autonomy" of A/A vaccines versus "conventional" vaccines, here it will be presented as an overview of the necessary points to consider, to guarantee an acceptable standard in the development and control of this particular category of veterinary immune-biologicals.

INTRODUCTION

Two fundamental issues must be preliminarily considered to proceed further with a critical review of the current state of the art of A/A vaccines, and to hypothesise about future scenarios in their production and control. First of all, it must be recognized that the need for promoting a specific debate about this category of veterinary immune-biologicals, originates from the circumstance that they are out of the scope of any European Union (EU) codification and, as a consequence, each Member State can control these products by its own regulation. The lack of a harmonized approach within and among Member States can create a number of controversial situations. Secondly, it must be agreed that these products are worthy of interest. Although A/A vaccines are generally considered of less scientific value compared to "conventionally codified" ("conventional») vaccines, their production has been historically admitted and the users have traditionally welcomed their use. In addition, several manufacturers of "conventional" vaccines are also involved and interested in the production of A/A vaccines. Once agreed that A/A vaccines are susceptible to interest, it should be possible to proceed with the recognition of this interest. The first step of such a process should focus on the formal evaluation of the characteristics of A/A vaccines (are they valuable products ?), and should lead to the acceptance of their "status" from a regulatory and scientific point of view. The next steps should allow the functional characterization of A/A vaccines (do they fulfil a useful function ?) and the establishment of specific rules for their production and control. The whole process, although assessing the autonomy of A/A vaccines, should allow the development and use of safe and efficacious A/A vaccines, and indirectly "protect" the regulatory status of "conventional» vaccines.

The Process for Recognizing Interests of Autologous/Autogenous Vaccines: How Regulation and Science Should Allow Formal and Functional Acceptance of A/A Vaccines

The provisions and requirements relating to the authorisation of veterinary medicinal products in the EU are laid down in Directive 2001/82/EC of 6/11/01 [1] and in Council Regulation (EEC) 2309/93 of 22/7/93 [2]. Several points in the two codifications are of interest for carrying out the process of formal evaluation of A/A vaccines. In the introductory remarks of the directive, the concepts of "harmfulness" and "therapeutic efficacy" (point 11), of "pharmaco-vigilance" — safety (point 27) and "pharmacovigilance" — lack of efficacy — (point 29) are mentioned. Article 1, points 7 defines an immunological veterinary medicinal product (IVMP), whereas points 10, 13 and 16 introduce, respectively, the concepts of adverse reaction, unexpected adverse reaction and off-label use. Article 2 establishes the field of application of directive 2001/82/EC and defines the concept of marketing authorization (MA) "inter alia". Whereas art. 3, point 2 introduces the concept of A/A vaccines, art. 4, point 1 establishes a formal difference between inactivated and non-inactivated A/A vaccines. Furthermore, point 2 in the same article introduces some exemptions in the authorization of vaccines for minor species. Part B of the Council Regulation introduces the concepts of medicinal products presented for an entirely new indication which in the opinion of the European Agency for the Evaluation of Medicines (EMEA) is of significant therapeutic effect (point 3), and of veterinary medicinal products intended for use in food producing animals containing a new active substance which on the date of entry into force of the regulation, was not authorized by any Member State for use in food-producing animals (point 8). On the basis of regulatory limits posed by the Directive, "conventional" vaccines are those immune-biologicals holding an MA "inter alia" and a full dossier has to be submitted for obtaining it. Minor Use/Minor Species (MUMS) vaccines should generally hold an MA but reduced requirements are needed for submission of the dossier of registration. A/A vaccines do not need an MA. Table 1 summarizes the regulatory limits which apply to these three categories of veterinary immune-biologicals.

Table 1: Regulatory limits of "Conventional" and A/A vaccines.

Conventional vaccines MA inter alia	**MUMS vaccines MA inter alia**	**A/A Vaccines No MA**

• Full dossier	• Reduced requirements
	• Applicable to:
	  • Minor use
	  • Minor species
		• Reduced requirements
		• Restricted use in terms of the number of animals treated
		• No limit if
		  • Minor use
		  • Minor species

Whereas no limit in the species of destination or in the indication of use is applied, restriction in terms of the number of treated animals is requested. Reduced requirements for the submission of the protocols of production and control are allowed. In particular, whereas quality and safety documentation should be similar for "conventional" MUMS and A/A vaccines, characteristics of efficacy could vary. "Conventional" and MUMS vaccines are in fact administered for prophylactic purposes and their efficacy is demonstrated through a model of preventive vaccination of the animals followed by an experimental challenge. A/A vaccines can be applied in the case of continuing infections, either for "therapeutic" (autologous vaccines) or for "metaphylactic" purposes (autogenous vaccines). Their efficacy is only "presumed" (a continuing infection is followed by vaccination of animals). Regulatory limits have to be respected to avoid confusion (e.g. between MUMS and A/A vaccines), fraudulent use (e.g. escaping MA, extended use of A/A vaccines to a larger number of animals and conditions) and intermediate markets (e.g. "experimental" use). As far as the Council Regulation is concerned, confusion or contradictory situations could be generated by applying the same concepts of new indications (e.g. "therapeutic" effect) and new substance (e.g. strain/antigen specificity). Based on these specific aspects, the same IVMP could be considered as A/A vaccine (no MA) or eligible for a centralized procedure (either mandatory, part A or, optionally, part B).

By definition, autologous vaccines have been historically used to treat "chronic" infectious diseases of single animals. For our purposes, "continuing infection" should replace the significance of "chronic" disease, and the terms "therapeutic" vaccine or "pharmavaccine" could replace "autologous" vaccine. To adopt these terms, it appears necessary to define the significance of "therapeutic" effect applied to a veterinary vaccine and, if possible, to demonstrate the efficacy of a "therapeutic" vaccine. Indeed, such a concept is better applied to major categories of human medicinal products which are used in conditions where there is a malfunction of the immune-system (e.g. allergies, auto-immune diseases and cancer). Nevertheless, considering the lack of experimental data in animals, it could be assumed that a "therapeutic" veterinary vaccine can, at least, influence the course of the disease (e.g. by allowing a quicker recovery or healing of lesions, such as in papillomatosis).

By contrast, whether or not a "therapeutic" vaccine can be considered efficacious or influence the eradication of the causative agent of a specific disease (and in this case it could be interesting to investigate the effector mechanisms of the immune-system involved in such a process), remains questionable.

By definition, autogenous vaccines have been historically used to treat continuing infections of animals present in a holding (equivalent terms are "stable" or "herd" vaccines). The treatment of continuing infections (the unexpected event represents the rationale for the use of autogenous vaccines) is based on the selection of well characterized strains/antigens with the aim of developing extremely specific vaccines. As for autologous vaccines, the antigenic specificity of immune-protective "therapeutic" or" metaphylactic" vaccination is difficult to demonstrate. In consideration of such a difficult task, the current "misuse" of autogenous vaccines as a preventive, prophylactic tool in the herd of origin, remains a crucial aspect from the regulatory point of view. While the treatment of animals in the case of continuing infection could directly result in the eradication of the causative agent, indirect effects could be represented by an aid in recovering animal performances, reducing losses, etc. In addition, targeted therapy or the use of vaccines for biological therapy, are relatively new issues worth considering when discussing novel approaches to the use of autogenous vaccines. In these cases, the respect of individual autonomy (including the professional autonomy of the veterinarian or the private autonomy of the possible counterparts, such as farmers) which allows for the freedom to choose independently either a therapy or a prophylaxis (e.g. biological therapy applied to replace the use of antibiotics) should be taken into account. Finally it is worth mentioning the necessity of avoiding the potential paradox inherent in the concepts of antigen specificity and immune-specificity (common characteristics of both "high tech" and autogenous vaccines). The need for extreme specificity could lead to the development either of "high tech" vaccines (mainly viral vaccines), or of autogenous vaccines (mainly bacterial vaccines): in one case an MA obtained through a mandatory centralized procedure in the EU is needed; in the case of an autogenous vaccine no MA is needed (be aware of consistency with Council Regulation (EEC) 2309/93). Table 2 compares specific features of prophylactic, metaphylactic and therapeutic effects of "conventional" and A/A vaccines.

Table 2: Prophylactic/Methaphylaxis/Therapeutic effects of vaccines.

	Prophylaxis	**Metaphylaxis**	**Therapeutic effect**
Use	Preventive	Continuing infections	Continuing infections
Alternative Use	Never continuing infections	Preventive ?	Never preventive !
Strain/Antigen	Standard	Herd-specific	Animal-specific
Immunity	**Conventional vaccine** Wide spectrum	**Autogenous vaccine** Mainly local and specific	**Autologous vaccine** ?
Result	Efficacy	Treatment of symptoms + indirect effects (i.e. help in recovering animal performances)	Local treatment + indirect effects (i.e., quicker recovery or healing of lesions)

FUTURE PERSPECTIVES AND PROPOSALS

After having agreed on the useful function of A/A vaccines, the next step should allow the setting of appropriate rules capable of guaranteeing the use of safe and efficacious products. The widest consensus among the different parties involved in the process of recognition of A/A vaccines is envisaged and should be reached. It would be advisable to continue promoting regulatory and scientific debates to clearly differentiate between the categories of A/A vaccines in respect to "conventional» vaccines. Furthermore, the magnitude of the phenomenon should be acknowledged by conducting a survey of the type of products, number of doses produced and sold, e.g. in the past three to five years, of diagnostic centres, approved manufacturers and regulatory conditions (including pharmaco-vigilance issues) in each Member State. Studies finalized to improve the knowledge of A/A vaccines (e.g. investigation of metaphylactic and therapeutic effects) or to develop study models (mode of action and efficacy control) should be envisaged. For the setting of rules, it appears necessary to define and harmonize major characteristics of A/A vaccines (e.g. to adopt more specific terminology, allow only inactivated A/A vaccines to be used, avoid the use of viral A/A vaccines unless extremely justified), to select and harmonize specific criteria for using A/A vaccines (e.g. allow their use only under unexpected events, do not allow a massive use or their use in farms other than the originating one, do not allow their use if commercial alternatives exist). In any case the use of A/A vaccines should be subordinated to a justification for the specific use and to a risk/benefit analysis. Responsibilities must be unequivocally recognized and attributed (e.g. veterinarians, diagnostic laboratories, production centres, farmers), and in addition, the traceability of the products must be guaranteed. Finally, it would be advisable to prepare guidelines to evaluate the quality, safety and efficacy of A/A vaccines.

A/A vaccines should be produced exclusively under the approval of competent national authorities of facilities, personnel, documents and production outlines/SOPs. Although keeping regulatory requirements reduced in respect of "conventional» vaccines, a minimum standard in production should be established. Harmonization of the registration of production records, production procedures (e.g. establishing inactivating agent concentration, limits for adjuvants, parameters for sterility and safety testing, etc.), and of labelling, should be enforced.

Veterinarians and diagnostic laboratories are the figures involved in the preliminary phase of the production. The request for any A/A vaccine can only be certified by a veterinarian. Diagnostic centres then proceed with the isolation, identification and characterization of the pathogen. The production centre will then be responsible for the preparation of the A/A vaccine. A rationale for the production must be presented, as well as a description of the equipment, starting materials, reference standards and package materials. The whole process of production and control must be described. Production and control steps should include initial testing of purity of master seeds and cell lines, growing the micro-organism, testing its identity and purity, inactivating the micro-organism, testing for inactivation, formulation of the vaccine preparation, blending and bottling, controls of the finished product (including physical-chemical tests, e.g. appearance, pH, volume, density, assays of the adjuvants and inactivating agents, sterility, safety and potency, e.g. antigen load-testing). A minimum of indications is required in the package insert (e.g. dose, route of administration, vaccination schedule). Finally, collection of data from the field to ensure target animal safety and efficacy, and registration of the results obtained for each batch of any A/A vaccines used in a farm, should be realized.

References

1 Directive 2001/82/EC of the European Parliament and of the Council of 6 November 2001 on the Community code relating to veterinary medicinal products. Official Journal of the European Communities, 28.11.2001 L 311/1-L 311/66.

2 Council Regulation (EEC) 2309/93 of 22 July 1993 laying down Community procedures for the authorization and supervision of medicinal products for human and veterinary use and establishing the European Agency for the Evaluation of Medicinal Products. Journal of the European Communities, 21.8.1993 L 214/1-L214/21.

Dr. M. Tollis, Istituto Superiore di Sanità, Viale Regina Elena, 299, I-00161 Roma, Italy.
E-mail: m.tollis@iss.it

Jungbäck C (ed): Consideration of Alternative Licensing Procedures for Vaccines for Minor Species, Minor Indications and Autogenous/Autologous Products.
Dev Biol. Basel, Karger, 2004, vol 117, p 61.

SESSION I (Part 3)

Autogenous/Autologous Vaccines

Actual Situation and Handling in the Field: Producers' and Users' Point of View

Moderator: *B. Bönisch* (Merial)

Jungbäck C (ed): Consideration of Alternative Licensing Procedures for Vaccines for Minor Species, Minor Indications and Autogenous/Autologous Products.
Dev Biol. Basel, Karger, 2004, vol 117, pp 63-67.

Autogenous Vaccines: Current Use Patterns and End Users' Needs in the Integrated Broiler Industry

J.A. Smith

Fieldale Farms Corp., Baldwin, GA, USA

Only 0.18% of all doses of animal vaccines, bacterins, and vaccine/bacterin combinations produced in U. S. licensed establishments in 2002 were classified as autogenous products [1]. Nevertheless, autogenous vaccines and bacterins are increasingly important adjuncts to health maintenance and food safety in the integrated broiler, turkey, and egg industries in the U. S. A survey was submitted to the three major producers of autogenous poultry vaccines in the U. S. These three producers manufactured in 2002 approximately 105,000,000 doses of roughly 100 different autogenous vaccines and bacterins for 78 customers. At least 16 different species of organisms were used, including *Bordetella avium, Erysipelothrix rhusiopathiae, E. coli, Haemophilus paragallinarum, Mycoplasma spp., Ornithobacterium rhinotracheale, Pasteurella multocida, Riemerella anatipestifer, Salmonella spp., Staphylococcus aureus,* Adenovirus, Avian Influenza Virus, Infectious Bronchitis Virus, Infectious Bursal Disease Virus, Avian Paramyxovirus 3, and Reovirus. Customers included primary broiler and turkey breeder companies, broiler and turkey integrators, and table egg producers.

The need for autogenous vaccines seems to be increasing. There are four main factors driving this need.

The Pathogens

Many of the major pathogens have a demonstrated ability to mutate and drift antigenically. Infectious Bursal Disease (IBD), Infectious Bronchitis Virus (IBV), and Reovirus are prominent examples. Today's vertically integrated poultry business structure has resulted in dense poultry populations that turn over rapidly.

Large, changing poultry populations probably contribute to the rapid emergence of variant strains of these mutable viruses, driving the need for new vaccines. Widespread use of commercial vaccines applies selection pressure, encouraging the survival of mutants that are different from the commercial vaccine strains. The immense size and wide geographical distribution of the industries create the possibility for geographically localized variants as well.

The Host

The birds have been selected intensively for productive characteristics, and as a result experience considerable physiological stress associated with rapid growth. Stress reduces innate resistance and adaptive immune responses. Relatively minor antigenic changes in a pathogen, that may have gone undetected years ago, are now resulting in measurable decreases in productivity and even overt disease in these modern, rapidly growing and heavily laying birds. Practitioners working with today's genetics need vaccines that are more closely matched antigenically to the resident pathogens. The increased fragility of the modern bird is especially evident in heavy breeder males, which have been selected most intensively of all. These males tolerate live *P. multocida* vaccines poorly, and so the reliance on killed fowl cholera vaccines has increased. The extreme serotype specificity of killed fowl cholera vaccines has necessitated widespread use of autogenous fowl cholera vaccines for the local serotypes in cockerels.

New Management Priorities

Couple this increased sensitivity of the modern host with efforts to decrease the use of antimicrobials, and the need for rigorous, precise prophylactic strategies is apparent. Food safety and salmonella control are increasingly important. With over 2,400 serovars, autogenous salmonella vaccines are critical to advancing salmonella control, especially in primary and multiplier breeders.

The Vaccine Industry

The commercial vaccine industry is becoming concentrated in fewer, larger businesses, and the process for regular (as opposed to autogenous or conditional) licensing of a commercial vaccine is rigorous, as it should be. Unfortunately this structure is not exceedingly nimble. It is difficult to respond quickly to a new pathogen with a regularly licensed product. The poultry vaccine business is also extremely competitive, with narrow profit margins that depend on volume for profitability. It is not economically feasible to respond to a geographically localized pathogen with a regularly licensed product. If either a new or a geographically localized pathogen becomes permanently established and widespread, then a regularly licensed commercial product is feasible and should be required. In the meantime, autogenous vaccines are the better alternative.

The U.S. regulations governing the manufacture of autogenous vaccines in 9 CFR 113.113 are administered by the United States Department of Agriculture, Animal and Plant Health Inspection Service, Veterinary Services, Center for Veterinary Biologics (the agency). While these regulations have served the veterinary profession and the regulatory agency well, they no longer fully meet the needs of the modern commercial poultry industry. Commercial poultry veterinarians who are the end users of these vaccines have approached the agency via the American Association of Avian Pathologists' (AAAP) Biologics Committee with several specific concerns.

The regulations apparently were devised with individual cattle and swine herds and private practitioners in mind. It apparently was assumed that autogenous vaccines would be used primarily to address sudden, severe outbreaks of livestock disease, usually in a single herd or in a localized area. Once the outbreak was quelled, the need for the vaccine should disappear. Autogenous vaccines are no longer used solely to control sudden epornitics. Due to the changes in the industry, in the birds, and in disease prevention priorities, autogenous products are used in a truly prophylactic manner. "Less-than-serotype" changes in mutable and emerging viruses are followed much more closely than in the past, to control diseases as they emerge, not after they are out of hand. Some practitioners use commercial vaccines as the basis of their immunization programmes, with additional autogenous vaccines that evolve as the pathogens evolve, literally one step behind the pathogens. We are attempting to provide the most homologous protection possible, to minimize disease and our reliance on antimicrobials as far as possible.

It would appear that there has been (and perhaps remains) a need to protect the farmer from unscrupulous veterinarians and vaccine manufacturers, and to prevent unscrupulous manufacturers from using the autogenous regulations to circumvent the process of obtaining full licensing for some products. These safeguards need to remain in place. However, the current structure of the poultry industries (broilers, turkeys, and layers) is such that some of these safeguards are not only no longer needed, but are actually interfering with effective use of autogenous products. The integrated company owns the parent breeder birds and retains ownership of the production progeny. Most of the larger companies have staff veterinarians who are full-time employees of the company. In terms of the veterinarian-client-patient relationship, the veterinarian-employee is a part of the client, and the patients are his employer's animals. These veterinarians are typically poultry specialists, and are quite capable of assessing the field safety and efficacy of the vaccines they use. The tight profit margins in the poultry industries preclude the use of any product, including a vaccine, which does not appear to give a return. If a veterinarian employed by an integrator is using worthless vaccines, the problem is between that veterinarian and his employer, not between the manufacturer and the integrator. The prospects of a shyster foisting a worthless product on an unsuspecting or uneducated user are unlikely. Today, an unaffiliated practitioner or a vaccine manufacturer does not approach the owners of poultry flocks (the integrators) with an offer to make an autogenous vaccine to solve a purported problem. Rather, the corporate veterinarian has identified the problem, determined the need for an autogenous vaccine, and approaches the manufacturer with a well-characterized organism in hand, asking the manufacturer to produce the vaccine for his operation. Given the resources and time, corporate veterinarians and consultants could legally produce these vaccines in their own laboratories for use in their own birds. It is preferable to have competent, experienced manufacturers produce them under commercial manufacturing practices. The regulations should foster this relationship, not hinder it, and could be modified to allow more efficient use without compromising prudent regulatory control.

Four specific concerns have been articulated by various members of the AAAP Biologics Committee. The first two were endorsed and sent forward to the agency by the Committee. The second two remain concerns of some individuals.

1. The regulations require that an autogenous vaccine be used only in the herd from which the organism was isolated [9 CFR 113.113 (a) (2) and (a) (3)], and impose extensive application procedures for use in adjacent and non-adjacent herds. The agency has been fairly liberal in interpreting this part of the regulation in terms of commercial poultry flocks. The special structures of the integrated industries (whether broilers, turkeys, layers, swine, or others) should be recognized and acknowledged in the regulation, rather than depending on the interpretation of future administrators. The structure of integrated operations makes the criteria in paragraph (a) (3) (iii) a permanent and continuing feature. The integrated structure, by its very nature, always ensures that the "epidemiology of the disease situation… links the designated geographical areas with the herd (i.e. flock) of origin…" An autogenous vaccine produced for any flock within an integrated production complex should be available for use anywhere in that complex.

2. The regulations limit vaccine production to 15 months from the original isolation, or 12 months from the production of the first serial, whichever comes first. Additional serials may be produced for up to 24 months upon presentation of supporting information to the Administrator, including a "documentation of continued involvement". Extension beyond 24 months requires antigenicity and potency tests. These additional safeguards are not needed. If the vaccine is effective, it should be difficult or impossible to re-isolate that pathogen or otherwise "document continued involvement". It is quite possible and in many cases likely that the pathogen remains a threat. Under the current guidelines, the practitioner must stop vaccinating, allow some flocks to fall sick, re-isolate the pathogen, and start again. If the pathogen has indeed disappeared, and the autogenous product is no longer needed, where is the real harm in the integrated system ? There are probably no adverse effects whatsoever on the birds, farmers, or consumers from continued use of the vaccine. The only disadvantage is the possibility of money ill-spent on an unnecessary vaccine, and informed individuals who own the birds and stand the loss will have evaluated the risks and made the decision to continue use.

3. Some practitioners desire the ability to add an autogenous antigen to existing standard antigens. There are several rational reasons for doing this, including a spectrum of protection and bird handling and stress. Mixing of separately prepared preparations in the field is fraught with numerous dangers, such as contamination, incompatibility of emulsions, and homogeneous distribution of components. A combination of autogenous and regularly licensed antigens by the manufacturer should be permitted. Appropriate testing of the regularly licensed fraction could be conducted as usual.

4. It is unclear whether a manufacturer can return an isolate to the owner. It is clear that isolates must be destroyed after the allowed 12 to 15 months (or 24-month

extension). Some practitioners desire clear permission to retrieve isolates. The inability to do so precludes the ability to switch manufacturers, is an unnecessary restraint of commerce, and denies access to what is regarded as proprietary ownership of the isolate. If the time limits were to be rescinded as suggested, there should be no reason that an isolate could not be returned.

The objectives should be to produce autogenous vaccines that are pure and safe, and that meet the challenges of emerging or localized diseases, within a regulatory framework that maintains adequate regulatory control while recognizing the current structure of the industries.

Reference

1 USDA APHIS VS CVB, Ames, IA 50010-8197. Veterinary Biologics Notice No. 70. Veterinary biological products in licensed establishments produced and destroyed 01/01/02 through 12/31/02.

Dr. J.A. Smith, MAM, Fieldale Farms Corp., PO Box 558, Baldwin, GA 30511, USA.
E-mail: johnsmith@fieldale.com

Jungbäck C (ed): Consideration of Alternative Licensing Procedures for Vaccines for Minor Species, Minor Indications and Autogenous/Autologous Products.
Dev Biol. Basel, Karger, 2004, vol 117, pp 69-71.

Autogenous Vaccines: Current Use in the Field in the U.S. Cattle and Hog Industry

C.C.L Chase

Department of Veterinary Science, South Dakota State University, Brookings, SD, USA

Autogenous vaccines are one of the tools of swine and bovine preventative health programmes. They fill a void when new agents emerge for which there are no vaccines or when antigenic variation occurs that is outside the spectrum of protection afforded by commercially available vaccines. They have shown tremendous value in filling these gaps or in cases when diagnostic and molecular workups of isolates have shown there is a need for a different antigen. However at other times autogenous vaccines have been touted as a panacea or "miracle cure" and the answer to all problems without any basis in fact.

Autogenous vaccines have been used extensively for the past 20 years. In the swine industry, they were valuable for the control of atrophic rhinitis and colibacillosis in swine before the advent of efficacious commercial products. In the last few years, they have been important for the control of porcine reproductive and respiratory syndrome (PRRSV) and swine influenza. They are being used for circoviruses because of the lack of any commercial vaccines. With PRRSV and swine influenza, their greatest value has been when extensive diagnostic and molecular techniques have been used to differentiate between the field strains which were different from those organisms in commercial vaccines. This science-based application of autogenous vaccines is tremendously important for preventative swine health. In cattle, autogenous vaccines have not been as widely used. They have been used to prevent infections with *Mycoplasma bovis, Mannheimia (Pasturella) haemolytica* and *Morexella bovis* to name just a few pathogens that have been incorporated into bovine autogenous vaccines.

As a food animal veterinarian and veterinary microbiologist, what do I see as the advantages of autogenous vaccines? The first is strain selection. Herd-specific strains can be used. These strains have often been analysed molecularly and shown to be antigenically different from commercial vaccines strains. Secondly, there is the ability to select specific adjuvants depending on whether an antibody or cell-mediated response is needed. Finally, formulations can be developed that increase the amount of antigen and also antigen combinations can be used.

What is the disadvantage of autogenous vaccines? The first is efficacy testing; commercial vaccines must use a challenge model with the pathogenic organism and prove that the vaccine protects against disease. The ability to deliver autogenous vaccines quickly to the producer for newly emerging diseases, the major reason for autogenous vaccines, is a double-edged sword; the vaccine is available, but will it work? Just because a vaccine contains an organism, there is no guarantee that it will protect. What about adventitious agents in autogenous vaccines? Although all autogenous vaccines in the U.S. must be inactivated, contamination of a viral vaccine with another virus such as bovine herpesvirus 1 [BHV-1, infectious bovine rhinotracheitis (IBR)] could result in animals being sero-positive for diseases that have been eradicated in other countries and these vaccinated animals would not be eligible for export. The only testing requirement for USDA-approved autogenous vaccines is safety. Safety is only required by USDA for those companies that produce for interstate sale and is likely only in those few companies who also produce USDA-licensed products in addition to autogenous products. A third problem is access to new generation adjuvants. One of the major developments in the vaccine industry in the last 10 years is new adjuvants. In the past, the major concern in vaccine development was the organism. The adjuvant was just an afterthought. These new adjuvants make previously "poor" vaccine antigens like *Mycoplasma hyopneumoniae* highly effective. Most of these adjuvants are proprietary and are available only in commercial vaccines. These new adjuvants require extensive testing to ensure that they do not cause side effects such as adverse reactions or abscess. The proprietary nature and the cost of testing limits the availability of these adjuvants for autogenous vaccines and results in the use of less efficacious adjuvant formulations in autogenous vaccines. The final problem is the lack of interference testing of multiple antigen products that contain *Mycoplasma hyopneumoniae.* Clients like to minimize the number of vaccinations, but certain antigens may require different types of adjuvants and the antigens in these combinations can be antagonistic rather than synergistic. In my experience this has been a particular problem with *Mycoplasma hyopneumoniae* combination vaccines as they give little protection against *Mycoplasma hyopneumoniae.*

As a practitioner, I am a proponent of autogenous vaccines when used prudently. In clinical practice, we produced many autogenous rhinitis vaccines before the introduction of efficacious commercial vaccines, that were highly effective at controlling rhinitis in our clients' herds. These herds were cultured routinely and slaughter checks were performed to assess the efficacy of the vaccine programme. When commercial rhinitis vaccines became available, we were able to switch to these vaccines. Autogenous vaccines account for 15-20% of the U.S. swine market and are likely to double in the next 10 years as the swine industry becomes more integrated. Autogenous usage in the cattle industry is much lower but also will probably increase as veterinarians and producers continue to improve preventative health programmes.

Initiating a preventative health programme without any monitoring programme to assess the outcome of the vaccine programme is like shooting in the dark. One of the biggest problems in the field is "consultants" for autogenous companies who have actively solicited clients to produce an autogenous vaccine by promising that an autogenous vaccine would cure their "problems". This was without any diagnostic preparation, but an "over-the-fence" diagnosis. In almost all cases these units had multiple management problems; the idea that the answer to all problems comes out of the end of a needle is ridiculous. Vaccines are only a part of most disease prevention programmes. In swine *Streptococcus suis* has frequently been the major target of these "miracle vaccines". Finding a "protective vaccine" for *Strep. suis* will require a subunit vaccine and an excellent adjuvant that will probably require commercial development. The other major autogenous vaccine misuse is developing vaccines for organisms that rarely cause disease. These types of vaccines are just a "cure" looking for a disease. Statements that the autogenous vaccine is "just like" company X's but is 10¢ a dose cheaper are often just market-driven without any efficacy data. One production unit in our practice used a bargain *Mycoplasma hyopneumoniae* autogenous vaccine. This unit developed a recurrent cough and had extensive Mycoplasma lesions on slaughter check. This cost "saving" was a real loser to this unit.

When should autogenous vaccines be used on a swine or cattle production operation? First, the use of any vaccine should be science-based. That means diagnostic preparation was done and the organism and a production problem (reproductive, performance, etc.) was identified. Only finding an organism without any evidence of disease or production problems does not automatically mean we need to control or prevent that organism with a vaccine. Second, if no commercial vaccine is available and the herd health veterinarian feels an autogenous vaccine is the right approach, contact autogenous manufacturers for cost and minimum order requirements. Contact companies should be those who produce commercial USDA-approved biologicals because they will most probably have adopted many of the quality control/quality assurance standards from their commercial production for their autogenous production. Third, if a commercial product is available and has not performed to expectations, contact the commercial company. If the herd health veterinarian feels there is no remedy from a commercial vaccine, an autogenous vaccine may be the solution. Again the organism needs to be re-isolated and extensive diagnostic laboratory evaluation (including genetic analysis) performed to determine that the organism is different from commercial vaccine antigens. Fourth, if a new commercial product becomes available for the disease agent against which the autogenous vaccine was developed, a vaccine trial comparing the autogenous to the new product should be run. With the new adjuvants and vaccine technologies, the majority of the time the commercial vaccine will be superior to the autogenous vaccine. Finally, do not let the cost of the vaccine alone be the major factor in selecting an autogenous vaccine over a commercial vaccine. If a complete economic evaluation looking at performance, morbidity and mortality is not done for the vaccine, the true savings or loss will not be known. Always let science and the economic bottom line guide whether an autogenous vaccine is used, not emotions or someone else's persuasive skills.

Dr. C. Chase, Department of Veterinary Science, ADRDL Bldg, Rm. 125, Box 2175, South Dakota State University, Brookings, SD 57007, USA
E-mail: christopher_chase@sdstate.edu

Jungbäck C (ed): Consideration of Alternative Licensing Procedures for Vaccines for Minor Species, Minor Indications and Autogenous/Autologous Products.
Dev Biol. Basel, Karger, 2004, vol 117, pp 73-81.

Current Situation and Use of Autogenous Vaccines in France: The Views of the Manufacturer and the User

E. Thibault

Biovac, Beaucouze, France

INTRODUCTION

The veterinary use of autogenous vaccines, products originally developed by veterinarians themselves, has grown over the past twenty years. The causes are many: the emergence of new diseases, better diagnosis, the existence of laboratories specializing in autogenous vaccine production, and the expectations of society and economic constraints, which prefer prevention to cure.

Despite this, the use of autogenous vaccines is limited and the lack of information given to veterinarians does not explain everything. This document is intended to describe the situation in France with regard to the use of autogenous vaccines and to describe the expectations of both the manufacturer and the prescribing veterinarian user.

THE CURRENT SITUATION

Today's situation results partly from current regulations and partly from the efficacy, cost and availability of licensed vaccines.

Regulatory bases

Autogenous vaccines are defined in article L.5141-2 of the French Code of Public Health (Code de la Santé Publique — CSP): « *By an autogenous vaccine for veterinary use is meant any immunological veterinary medicine manufactured with the aim of inducing active immunity using pathogenic organisms obtained from one or more animal(s) in a single herd, that have been inactivated and used to treat an animal or animals from the herd».* This article therefore specifies the conditions of use of the autogenous vaccine, which can only be used for the herd in which the pathogenic agent was discovered that has been incorporated into the vaccine.

Article L.5141-12 of the CSP specifies the conditions for the granting of authorization to manufacture autogenous vaccines: *«The preparation of autogenous vaccines for veterinary use must be carried out by a qualified person who has obtained a permit from the French Veterinary Medicines Agency [l'Agence Nationale du Médicament Vétérinaire] for this purpose».*

While awaiting the appearance of an administrative order currently being compiled to amend the CSP, permits are limited to the manufacture of bacterial autogenous vaccines.

The current situation is therefore greatly influenced by regulatory requirements and the only drugs authorized, in practice, are bacterial autogenous vaccines used on the farm where the antigen(s) incorporated were isolated.

Efficacy, cost and availability of vaccines with an MA

The recognized **efficacy** of licensed vaccines justifies the preference for using products of this type instead of autogenous vaccines. Thus, more than 85 % of the 44 proprietary vaccine products available in France incorporating solely bacterial antigens are systematically preferred to an autogenous vaccine. A lack of efficacy was mentioned for only three of the seven products to which prescribers sometimes prefer an autogenous vaccine (Table 1).

Table 1: Bacterial vaccine or autogenous vaccine – selection criteria.

Bacterial vaccines	Choice of autovaccine: reasons			
	Efficacy	Combination with other antigens not present in the vaccine	Cost	Total
44	3	3	1	7

Despite the commonly held view, the **price** of a licensed vaccine in France is usually lower than that of an autogenous vaccine: this is, for instance, true of vaccines with indications for cattle, all of which are less expensive than an autogenous vaccine that would offer the same valences. Of the 44 proprietary products, price only emerges as the decisive factor in the choice of the autogenous vaccine in one, which is intended for racing and show pigeons (Table 1).

The **availability** of licensed vaccines is the main factor in the choice of the autogenous vaccine: thus, 85 % of the antigens introduced into the autogenous vaccines intended for poultry are not included in any of the licensed vaccines.

The place of autogenous vaccines in the veterinarian's medicine chest

The current situation of the French autogenous vaccines market, is characterized by the following features:

– Its **small size**: in a market that is estimated at 160 million €, **autogenous vaccines make up barely 2 % of all the commercial vaccines**.

- **Niche markets**: **minor species** and **secondary pathologies** make up the autogenous vaccine market. Furthermore, the « made to measure » manufacturing process means that the route of administration can be adapted to the species:
  (i) Autogenous vaccines for ducks and geese, guinea-fowl, pigeons, quails and game birds make up 60 % of the poultry autogenous vaccine production of our company;
  (ii) The diversity of antigens introduced in autogenous vaccines is high (Tables 2-5);

Table 2: Bacterial species included in autogenous vaccines for poultry.

Species	Serovariants and/or serotypes
Bacillus sphaericus	
Erysipelothrix rhusiopathiae	
Escherichia coli	O1, O2, O78 plus aerobactin strains +
Haemophilus sp	
Mannheimia haemolytica	
Pasteurella multocida	Numerous Heddleston and Namioka serotypes
Riemerella anatipestifer	A, G and 1 to 14.
Salmonella enterica	braenderup, derby, enteritidis (several lysotypes), hadar, heidelberg, infantis, kottbus, mbandaka, montevideo, newport, saintpaul, schwarzengrund, senftenberg, typhimurium (numerous lysotypes), virchow...
Staphylococcus aureus	
Yersinia pseudotuberculosis	

Table 3: Bacterial species included in autogenous vaccines for pigs.

Species	Biovars, serovariants and/or serotypes
Actinobacillus pleuropneumoniae	Biovars 1 and 2, serovars 2,3,4,6,7,8,9,11
Actinobacillus suis	
Actinomyces pyogenes	
Escherichia coli	18 serotypes commonly incorporated.
Haemophilus parasuis	2 dominant serovars
Pasteurella multocida	Serotypes A and D
Pseudomonas sp	
Salmonella enterica	
Staphylococcus aureus	
Staphylococcus hyicus	
Streptococcus bovis	
Streptococcus suis	Serotypes 1,1-2,2,3,4,5,6,7,8,9,10

Table 4: Bacterial species included in autogenous vaccines for fish.

Species	
Aeromonas salmonicida	*Photobacterium damselae* subsp. *piscicida*
Aeromonas sobria	*Renibacterium salmoninarum*
Flavobacterium psychrophilum	*Vibrio anguillarum*
Flexibacter maritimus	*Yersinia ruckeri*

Table 5: Bacterial species included in autogenous vaccines for ruminants.

Species	
Actinomyces pyogenes	*Staphylococcus chromogenes*
Bacillus cereus	*Staphylococcus epidermidis*
Brevibacterium sp	*Staphylococcus hominis*
Corynebacterium pseudotuberculosis	*Staphylococcus hyicus*
Enterobacter sp	*Staphylococcus intermedius*
Escherichia coli	*Staphylococcus schleiferi*
Haemophilus somnus	*Staphylococcus warneri*
Klebsiella pneumoniae	*Staphylococcus xylosus*
Mannheimia haemolytica	*Streptococcus agalactiae*
Microcoque de Morel	*Streptococcus bovis*
Moraxella bovis	*Streptococcus dysgalactiae*
Pasteurella multocida	*Streptococcus equisimilis*
Pasteurella trehalosi	*Streptococcus mutans*
Staphylococcus aureus	*Streptococcus sanguis*
Staphylococcus capitis	*Streptococcus uberis*
Salmonella enterica (abortusovis, calabar, heidelberg, infantis, montevideo, typhimurium…)	

(iii) Autogenous vaccines prepared specifically for the intra-dermal route achieve better vaccinal protection in rabbits (Table 6) and are effective in preventing infections resulting from the repeated use of the same needle in a herd of pigs.

Table 6: Influence of the route of administration on protection in rabbits.

Administration of an autogenous vaccine after six and eight weeks; challenge by intra-muscular injection of *P. multocida* at 10 weeks; mortality recorded for two weeks.			
Lot	**Unvaccinated control**	**Autogenous vaccine by sub-cutaneous route**	**Autogenous vaccine by intra-dermal route**
Antigens	—	*Pasteurella multocida* + *Bordetella bronchiseptica*	
Number of rabbits	19	19	18
Mortality	18	4	1
% mortality	**95 %**	**21 %**	**6 %**

- As a **response to needs not met** by the existing vaccines: autogenous vaccines are particularly indicated and prescribed for «**emerging diseases**» or in the context of a **lack of efficacy** of vaccines:
  (i) Many examples can be cited of the use of autogenous vaccines for new pathologies for which there are no vaccines in France: *Riemerella anatipestifer* infections in ducks (Table 7), Glässer's disease in pigs, mastitis due to *Streptococcus uberis* and *Staphylococcus aureus* in cattle, «pasteurellosis» due to *Mannheimia haemolytica* of serotypes not included in the vaccines for goats…

Table 7: Protection conferred by a *R. anatipestifer* autogenous vaccine in ducks.

Administration of the autogenous vaccine at three weeks of age; challenge by intra-muscular injection of *R. anatipestifer* at eight weeks.				
Results: mortality at 10 weeks (%)				
Experimental test	Number of birds/group	Unchallenged controls	Challenged controls	Autovaccinated birds
$0.6.10^6$	8	0	**8**	**0**
$0.4.10^4$	12	0	**12**	**0**
$0.8.10^6$	8	0	**8**	**0**

  (ii) In some situations in which the efficacy of a vaccine is called into question, an autogenous vaccine constitutes a pertinent alternative: for example this is the situation in avian pasteurellosis, for which the weakness of the cross protection induced by vaccine antigens does not always provide enough protection to prevent the onset of the disease (Table 8).

Table 8: P. multocida vaccines in ducks: assessment of the crossed protection.

Groups given the X73 Pm vaccine at five and seven weeks of age (V); Unvaccinated control lots (C); Challenge strains P. multocida serotype 1 (Heddleston's classification); Inoculation by intramuscular injection of 10^8 bacteria at nine weeks; mortality recorded for one week.										
Challenge strain	X73		A		B		C		D	
Group	C	V	C	V	C	V	C	V	C	V
Number of dead/ Total number	7/8	3/8	7/7	7/8	7/7	2/8	8/8	5/8	8/8	6/7
% mortality	87 %	38 %	100 %	**87 %**	100 %	25 %	100 %	62 %	100 %	**85 %**

- Sometimes **the extended use** relative to the guidelines of the regulatory use, at the initiative of the veterinarian: the definition of autogenous vaccines restricts their use to the herd from which the antigen included has been isolated; even though the definition of the «herd» is rather vague, this concept does not take into account how animal production is now organized (sectors for poultry, pigs and also for cattle or sheep for milk production and even fish farming), in which the flow of animals and of products (weekly deliveries of food, transfers of animals, twice-weekly collection of eggs and milk), the constant movements of people (farmers, technicians, intervention teams, veterinarians), lead to complex and major epidemiological links – and inevitably the related risks – that make the use of an autogenous vaccine within the limits specified by the present definition quite irrelevant.

In this context, **the veterinarian may feel the need to prescribe the use of an autogenous vaccine at places and for periods defined solely by the epidemiological ties uniting the animals vaccinated**. This is the case in the fight against pathogens of major importance for Public Health, such as *Salmonella typhimurium* in poultry or pig production, for instance: for the user, basic precaution demands that if a flock is contaminated in an animal-husbandry building, then it is necessary not only to vaccinate in the other buildings on the same farm, plus possibly the other production sectors on the farm, but also, and indeed above all, the other herds/flocks produced by the same organization, monitored by the same people, but spread over a much greater area than the original farm, and which are closely and permanently linked to this contaminated group. This precaution is dictated to the veterinarian by the necessity of controlling the identified epidemiological risk, and does not indicate the nature of the vaccine, be it a licensed vaccine or an autogenous one.

If a pathogen is so prevalent in a given type of production or within an organization that it is not possible to envisage slaughtering a contaminated herd, then vaccination, combined with draconian sanitary measures, is all the more appropriate because the risk of contamination is increased by keeping on the contaminated herd. In this context, **if the only vaccine available is an autogenous vaccine, it may become necessary to prescribe it on the scale of the company, using it beyond the regulatory framework, in herds and on farms where the pathogenic agent has not yet been isolated.**

What Future for Autogenous Vaccines?

The future of autogenous vaccines must take into account both the demands of society with regard to Animal Health and Public Health, and the constraints imposed on any economic sector. In practice, this means not leaving any animal disease without prevention on the one hand, and protecting the consumer on the other.

The use of autogenous vaccines is to be envisaged as a preference in the context of diseases for which there is no commercial vaccine. Consequently, the factors for the success of autogenous vaccines are, for the laboratory, the ability to produce a reliable product rapidly and for the prescribing veterinarian, the flexibility of use.

Prescription – Flexibility of use

The duty to care for animals is a fundamental principle in veterinary practice. In some cases, *this higher duty* may lead the veterinarian to prescribe an autogenous vaccine for use beyond its regulatory context; he or she must therefore *be able to justify* the reasons underlying his or her choice.

In the example of the fight against *S. typhimurium*, the application and use of an autogenous vaccine at the level of the breeder flocks that supply a duck hatchery led to the reduction in the percentage of excreting flocks, a reduction in the incidence of excretion in the contaminated flocks and an absence of contamination of the eggs laid (Tables 9-12). This is also true of contaminants other than *Salmonella*, but this is a particularly interesting case because it confronts the veterinarian with his/her responsibilities:

(i) the responsibility of the veterinarian who is acting outside the specified regulatory context;

(ii) the responsibility that arises from the duty of every veterinarian to promote the improvement of Public Health by reducing the risk of contamination and the presence of residues in food products;

(iii) the financial responsibility towards the company or organization that would face increased production costs if the farm is exposed to contamination or experiences an outbreak of disease.

Table 9: Protocol for monitoring the excretion of *S. typhimurium* in vaccinated and unvaccinated ducks breeding flocks.

Production cycle	Laying starts at 30 weeks; two laying periods lasting 20 to 22 weeks separated by a moult lasting 13 weeks.
Vaccination programme	Autogenous vaccine at 18, 22 and 27 weeks. Booster during the moult
Schedule of the tests carried out on each lot	Samples of dust and droppings taken from the farm every four weeks, i.e. five series per laying period.
	90 unfertilized eggs sampled every four weeks, i.e. five series per laying period.
Constitution of the lots	One out of two lots is vaccinated; all the lots included in the study are negative at 28 weeks of age.
Expression of the results	A lot is classified as positive if any sample is found to be positive; it is negative if all the results are negative

Table 10: S. typhimurium autogenous vaccine – positive flocks during the lay.

Positive/negative flocks		**Negative flocks**		**Positive flocks**	
		Number	**%**	**Number**	**%**
Autovaccinated flocks	46	37	**80 %**	9	20 %
Unvaccinated control flocks	42	24	57 %	18	**43 %**

Table 11: S. typhimurium autogenous vaccine – Degree of excretion of the contaminated flocks.

Frequency of positive samples in contaminated flocks		**Number of positive samples**			
		1		>1	
		Number	%	Number	%
Autovaccinated flocks	46	4	9 %	5	**11 %**
Unvaccinated control flocks	42	5	12 %	13	**31 %**

Table 12: S. typhimurium autovaccine – Flocks with infected eggs.

Flocks giving positive or negative egg samples		Negative flocks		Positive flocks	
		Number	%	Number	%
Autovaccinated flocks	46	46	**100 %**	0	0 %
Unvaccinated control flocks	42	32	76 %	10	**24 %**

This is the problem confronting responsible users: **veterinarians, who have to weigh up diverse imperatives – moral, regulatory and financial – and who assume liability as a result of their prescriptions and signatures, must be able to free themselves of an inappropriate definition of autogenous vaccines**, or else act to have it changed.

However, even though the definition that restricts the use of autogenous vaccines needs to be updated because it does not fit in with the demands of « modern » farming and the mobility that characterizes it, it would not be acceptable simply to get rid of the legislation that controls its production.

Manufacture – Reactivity and safety

The value of an autogenous vaccine for the veterinarian using it depends on how quickly it can be available in the context of a lack of commercial vaccines: for a Manufacturer adhering to Good Manufacturing Practice standard for veterinary medicines, the turn-around time cannot be less than four or even five weeks.

However, the legislation has not specified manufacturing standards, and so there are very considerable disparities between the manufacturers of autogenous vaccines. For instance, some manufacturers claim to be able produce an autogenous vaccine in under two weeks!

In France, the **preparation of autogenous vaccines is subject to obtaining a permit from the Ministries of Health and Agriculture**. In practice, fewer than 10 companies have received such a permit: most of them are not specialists but are diagnostic laboratories that have historically produced autogenous vaccines.

However, this **permit is not based on any standard or reference specifying manufacturing methods or control tests**: this deficiency is likely to lead to the preparation of dangerous products, that are inadequately inactivated and insufficiently tested, and to impair the long-term future of a product that is, in fact, very useful.

The French National Veterinary Medicines Agency is aware of the problem and is currently in the process of compiling draft legislation concerning autogenous vaccines for veterinary use in France, which specifies the conditions authorizing the preparation of these products. In particular, this text will define the qualification conditions and the scope of the responsibilities of the person qualified to prepare autogenous vaccines on the one hand, and the Good Manufacturing Practice standards for these products on the other.

As a corollary to the standardization of the manufacturing procedures and increased control of manufacturers, it should be possible to authorize the wider use of autogenous vaccines, under the supervision of the prescribing veterinarian, in specific circumstances and on condition that a pertinent rationale is provided.

The result of such measures would be the modification of the EEC order n°90/539, managing intra-EU exchanges of birds and eggs. Today, such birds have to be vaccinated with licensed vaccines only. For autogenous vaccines, in the case of their use under reinforced regulations and controls, there should be no reason to forbid exportation of birds vaccinated with these vaccines. And the word "licensed" of this order might be changed to "authorized".

In this context, the progressive introduction of tests and further checks could be envisaged depending on the number of animals vaccinated, based, for example, on the situation in the United States.

Conclusions

Autogenous vaccines are used in the context of an emergency or in the absence of a vaccine. As a result, the restrictions on their use are not readily accepted by prescribing veterinarians. In this context, it seems to be essential to standardize the manufacturing conditions for the production of autogenous vaccines in response to the needs of users and to guarantee their future as prescription-only veterinary products, intended for the prevention of infectious diseases in animals, within a regulatory framework that takes into account the epidemiological realities of animal husbandry.

Acknowledgements

The author would like to thank Doctor Jean Farges who clarified the rights and duties of veterinarians prescribing autogenous vaccines, and Doctor Daniel Gaudry for valuable advice while this document was being written.

Dr. E. Thibault, Biovac, 4 rue Olivier de Serres, B.P. 61, F-49071 Beaucouzé Cedex, France.
E-mail: biovac@biovac.fr

Jungbäck C (ed): Consideration of Alternative Licensing Procedures for Vaccines for Minor Species, Minor Indications and Autogenous/Autologous Products.
Dev Biol. Basel, Karger, 2004, vol 117, pp 83-86.

Manufacturing and Use of Autologous Vaccines in Germany – Experience of a Vaccine Manufacturer

A. Neubert

Impfstoffwerk-Dessau-Tornau GmbH, Rosslau, Germany

IDT produces commercial vaccines as well as herd- specific vaccines. The company was founded in 1921 and for a long period manufactured flock-specific products was one of the most important business areas. Interestingly, most of these vaccines were produced first for human use. One example was a sputum vaccine which was produced as a mixture of streptococci, staphylococci and pneumococci to prevent respiratory diseases in humans. Later more vaccines for veterinary use and herd-specific sera were manufactured. It is obvious that these herd-specific immunological products became more and more important and were used as powerful tools to treat or prevent infectious diseases. Some more historical examples are convalescent sera manufactured for ducks and geese, as well as live parapox ovis vaccines for goats and sheep.

Currently, with one exception, only inactivated bacterial vaccines are manufactured at a dedicated plant. The remaining viral product is a killed autologous papilloma virus vaccine used to treat infections in cattle, horses and dogs. The need for these products arose due to lack of efficient therapeutic or prophylactic means to cure these infections in farm animals. That situation has been made worse by the demand for reduced use of antibiotics and by the appearance of serotypes which are not included in commercial vaccines. Examples are avian colibacillosis, Staphylococci and Streptococci infections in pigs.

For rare diseases such as some Salmonella infections in various farm animals, game birds and exotic animals in zoos, immunological products are also very limited.

Furthermore one is faced with long duration and high costs for new developments and registration procedures which inhibit the elaboration of vaccines such as vaccines for Moraxella bovis infections or footrot in cattle.

It should also be mentioned that limited scientific knowledge of pathways and protective mechanisms of different infections may cause hurdles for development and licensing of vaccines. One example is the complex of reproductive disorders caused by Chlamydia in cattle.

In some of the cases described, the preparation and use of herd-specific vaccines can provide an efficient possibility to improve animal health in affected farms and flocks.

The most important feature before a vaccine can be produced is to analyse the situation on the farm and to obtain sufficient data about the disease. The disease and the hygienic conditions as well as stress factors should be evaluated and taken into consideration. It is necessary to have close contact with the veterinary service and to establish contact with diagnostic laboratories. The practitioners must receive all the information available about the possibilities and limitations of herd-specific vaccines for the disease. However, the most significant issue is to provide a reliable microbiological diagnosis. It is obvious that proper sampling procedures, well organised shipment and experienced laboratory staff are the most important topics for obtaining the right diagnosis.

One example is enterocolitis in suckling and feeding piglets. If only Clostridium perfringens, type A, was isolated, it could be a common organism which is found in the intestine in different species of animals. If further diagnosis identifies the beta 2 toxin-gene, it seems to be something different. In that case the isolate plays an aetiological role.

A formal order for a herd-specific vaccine including the microbiological data, the strain, species, quantity, location of the herd, address of the owner and the veterinarian needs to be transferred to the manufacturer.

In Germany there is no precise legislation for the manufacture of herd-specific vaccines. The Animal Disease Law (Tierseuchengesetz § 17 d) allows in general the preparation of herd-specific vaccines. The manufacturer needs general permission which allows him to produce all kinds of such vaccines. Some local administrations demand an overview at the end of the year which states what was produced.

Conditions for manufacturing are described in the Animal Vaccine Regulations (Tierimpfstoffverordnung). According to § 37 GMP conditions may not apply for herd-specific vaccines. The final decision can be made by the veterinary administration responsible for the federal state where the manufacturer is located. Furthermore general bio-safety regulations have to be considered. It seems to be obvious that the legislation for herd-specific vaccines is fragile. In comparison to the strict demands for licensed vaccines, it is necessary to compile a minimal set of regulations which considers the state-of-the – art for production and quality control of vaccines. However, the preparation of herd-specific vaccines needs higher flexibility hence GMP conditions cannot be applied.

The most significant quality issues rises with the use of starting material. These materials shall be free of extraneous agents and if possible be of pharmaceutical quality. Furthermore, residual limits need to be considered and if available only substances according to MRL regulation 2377/90/EEC Annex 2 without specified maximum residue limits shall be used. If substances according to Annex 1 are used, or local and systemic reactions occur, withdrawal periods shall be declared.

More critical and even impossible to investigate are contaminations hidden in the isolates. Sufficient information about the health status of the farm of origin and reliable inactivation procedures may overcome that issue. In fact it is more critical for viral vaccines than for bacterial products.

Reliable inactivation procedures means the method for the most resistant organisms and to check the inactivation for all batches with dedicated tests.

The preparation of a vaccine needs to be performed in conditions which are reproducible and described in written procedures. Written procedures need to be in place to ensure that the same procedures and manufacturing steps are followed.

The following table summarizes the minimum of in-process controls which are recommended for use in bacterial vaccines.

Table 1: Overview of in-process controls for manufacturing of herd-specific vaccines.

Manufacturing step	Test for purity	Test for pH	Test for CFU	Sterility	Toxicity in mice	Test for inactivation
Growth medium		+		+		
Strain	+					
Cultivation steps	+		+			
Inactivation				+	+ (for toxoid vaccines)	+
Bulk		+		+		

The determination of colony forming units (CFU) at the last step of fermentation is often the only possible way to define the antigen content of such a vaccine. There is a need to make more reliable tests available, such as antigen ELISA and Western blot assays. Controls on the filled vials should be scheduled to ensure the quality and consistency of the final vaccine.

It is considered necessary to provide results for the following quality parameters:

- Sterility
- Content of the inactivating agents (formaldehyde; BPL
- Concentration of preservatives (phenol, thiomersal)
- Content of the adjuvant (aluminium, oil)
- Pyrogenicity (Endotoxin/LAL test)

Specifications for endotoxin contents are difficult to set up. The knowledge of the toxicity of the bacterial endotoxin in the target species is often limited, but the data could help to investigate local or systemic side-effects.

There is a significant confusion which quality control methods shall be used. However, in general quality control tests described in the European Pharmacopoeia shall be used.

The shelf-life of a flock-specific vaccine is difficult to determine. It seems to be justified to put forward periods which are well established and investigated for comparable commercial vaccines. These vaccines are often based on the same starting materials and produced by the same way as herd-specific products. In that case commercial products can be used for up to 24 months and herd-specific vaccines shall be stable at least for a period of six months. That is considered as a minimal demand. The use of immunological products is based on vaccination of the complete flock including accrued animals. Hence the vaccine shall always be used for a longer period.

Beside manufacturing and quality issues it is most important to provide sufficient information to the veterinarian who is allocating the product. Comprehensive labels and informal instructions for use shall accompany the delivery of the vaccine.

The efficacy and safety of a herd-specific vaccine is much more than for commercial products predicted by good information practices. The manufacturer has acquired a set of data which can predict how reliably the vaccine can be used. That information shall be given to the practitioners and the farmer. For example, it is recommended that a new vaccine should always be tested on a small number of animals in the target herd. These tests cannot be omitted to prevent undesirable side effects. Often the animals are already affected by the disease and local or systemic reactions are much different than in naïve animals.

It should be pointed out that these vaccines shall always be directly applied by the veterinarian or at least under the control of the veterinarian. In that matter the regulations in Germany vary considerably; some Federal states have such demands that others do not.

The efficacy of herd-specific vaccines is much more difficult to follow up than safety. It is normally regulated by the market. If a product is efficient, it will be used again. The rising demand shows that the use of these products is desired and improves animal health even in difficult situations when no commercial product is available.

Nevertheless more sophisticated indicators for efficacy are much appreciated.

For a manufacturer of commercial vaccines the experience and epidemiological data gathered with herd-specific vaccines help to identify research strategies and could speed up the development of new products.

At IDT currently more than 21 species of bacterial organisms are used for the preparation of herd-specific vaccines. There are about 500 batches with about 6,000 litres of vaccines released per year.

Application of herd-specific vaccines is a versatile tool for the immunological control of animal diseases. The manufacturing and quality control shall be as close as possible to GMP and European Pharmacopoeia regulations. Starting materials and test methods shall be under control as well as for commercial vaccines.

In that direction the German legislation shall be revised to provide better support for manufacturing and application.

Dr. A. Neubert, Impfstoffwerk-Dessau-Tornau GmbH, Postfach 400214, D-06855 Rosslau, Germany.
E-mail: andreas.neubert@idt-direct.de

Jungbäck C (ed): Consideration of Alternative Licensing Procedures for Vaccines for Minor Species, Minor Indications and Autogenous/Autologous Products.
Dev Biol. Basel, Karger, 2004, vol 117, p 87.

SESSION II (Part 1)

Vaccines for Minor Use and Minor Species

Introduction, Producers' and Veterinarians' Point of View

Moderator: *D. Mackay* (Laboratory Institute for Animal Health)

Jungbäck C (ed): Consideration of Alternative Licensing Procedures for Vaccines for Minor Species, Minor Indications and Autogenous/Autologous Products.
Dev Biol. Basel, Karger, 2004, vol 117, pp 89-92.

Minor Species/Minor Indications – Introductory Remarks

C. Jungbäck

Paul-Ehrlich-Institut, Langen, Germany

The current European provisions concerning the licensing of vaccines do not provide exemptions for minor species/minor indications or rather minor use (MUMS) vaccines. Consequently, a lack of suitably authorised veterinary medicinal products in general and of vaccines in particular occurs. This is a problem both for animal welfare and for public health. In addition, the numerous mergers of manufacturers have led to a more global approach to market analysis. Therefore, the readiness to produce minor products for minor markets has decreased.

The purpose of this meeting is to take stock of the availability of vaccines intended for MUMS. The current legislation and the actual possibilities for placing MUMS products on the market should be analysed. In addition, pragmatic proposals to simplify administrative procedures should be developed and suggestions should be made on how to adapt scientific requirements to the essentials of MUMS vaccines. This meeting is dedicated explicitly to vaccines or, according to European vocabulary, to immunological veterinary medicinal products (IVMPs), because they are neglected in the current discussion on the availability of MUMS. The main part of the work already done on analyses and proposals for the availability of MUMS was performed for pharmaceuticals.

For pharmaceuticals, which are preferably used for therapeutical reasons, the MUMS problem is mainly reduced to the calculation of minimal residue limits (MRLs) of substances to ensure consumer protection.

Moreover, pharmaceuticals can be used throughout larger markets depending on the indication and/or the legal possibilities of veterinarians to widen the scope of animals to be treated, to use the cascade system, and to use products not or only exceptionally licensed. IVMPs are more difficult to handle. First, the species-specific variations in the immune system of various animals have to be taken into consideration. Cattle, sheep and goats are different in their immune reactions, even if closely related, and this is also the case for chickens and turkeys, geese, ducks, horses and donkeys, cats and lions and so on. Therefore the use of cascades should not be recommended for IVMPs.

The effect of vaccination cannot be controlled by means of observation of clinical parameters. Serological tests are necessary which may require sophisticated laboratory equipment and professional experience to obtain test results that provide reliable data.

The epidemiological relevance is the key item for the use of IVMPs and thus for the classification of a vaccine to be a MUMS product. The question whether an antigen is actually present in a certain area is a question not only of scientific but also of political interest. Vaccination will induce antibodies, which might disturb the diagnosis of field infections, block export possibilities, and influence the use of animals for breeding. Therefore, the need for a vaccine in a certain region has to be considered before the use of a MUMS-IVMP is licensed. In particular, live vaccines used in an area which is free of a certain disease and its antibodies, may set off an avalanche of induction of unwanted antibodies. The live antigen may induce recombination of new strains, which then affect larger regions and increase epizoological problems.

With respect to these items, the use IVMPs off label should be avoided. It will be much better to have licensed products available, the use of which is subject to official supervision and control. This is not the case with a large number of diseases and that is actually the crux of the matter.

First of all, a definition of MUMS is necessary, and I suppose this will not be very easy. Minor use is defined as a minor indication in a major species. Major species comprise a large number of animals and have a high economic impact. Minor diseases occur more or less rarely and are mainly of local importance. Minor species are defined by a threshold of animal numbers in a market and/or low economical value of the single animal. The crucial point for the definition of "minor" and "low" is to fix the relevant reference quantities.

The next decision to be made is how to approach MUMS. It would be useful to have a general definition for MUMS, but it may be impossible to define "major", "minor" or "low" precisely enough. An alternative for a definition may be a list of MUMS which will need permanent updating based on a harmonised approach. With respect to the European Union (EU) and its 25 Member States, it will certainly be a major and not a minor work to achieve a harmonised list of MUMS.

Another question to be answered is whether general requirements could be set or if case-by-case decisions may be necessary and then again, how to harmonise the latter within the EU.

The second step to facilitate the licensing of vaccines for MUMS necessitates a thorough assessment of the actual administrative, technical, and scientific requirements which have to be met by an applicant before being able to place an IVMP and especially a MUMS vaccine on the market.

For this purpose a number of items has to be considered:

Concerning administrative requirements, strong efforts should be made to simplify the procedures for licences and variations. As a number of MUMS-IVMPs may be regarded as being of public interest due to epizoological reasons in a certain region, the reduction or deletion of fees should be considered. Furthermore, the introduction of a legal instrument such as a conditional licence might be useful.

Currently, the EU legislation only allows impositions to be placed on a licence, an administrative instrument which is used very restrictively. It may also be essential to revise and, if necessary, reduce the so-called technical requirements such as Good Manufacturing Practice (GMP), Good Laboratory Practice (GLP) and Good Clinical Practice (GCP) for these products.

The pharmacovigilance system, created for products for human use, appears to be difficult to handle in the veterinary field, especially for MUMS products. In addition, the typical European problem of languages has to be solved. After the enlargement in 2004, we will have twenty-two languages within the EU. The translation of product literature into all official languages does not appear to be necessary for MUMS-IVMPs, even for centralised procedures. The EU Commission has stated that for EU-wide authorisations, translations in all twenty-two community languages will be obligatory. Here, a change of legislation appears to be inevitable to reach pragmatic solutions.

Concerning scientific requirements a large number of items may be considered for MUMS-IVMPs:

The expert reports in the dossier on quality, safety and efficacy should be questioned: Are these reports really necessary, could they be deleted or should they be modified from an overview of the dossier to risk-benefit assessments? Purity testing, especially extraneous agents testing, cannot be deleted, but it should be discussed whether the test systems required by EU regulations and European Pharmacopoeia (Ph. Eur.) monographs should be revised in a way to allow a larger range of test systems. In addition, replacement by other methods should be simplified not only for MUMS-IVMPs.

Following actual EU legislation including Ph. Eur., the safety test has to be performed with batches especially adjusted to the highest possible single dose. Vice versa, batches used for the performance of efficacy tests have to be adjusted to the lowest possible single dose. Here, it should be questioned whether the test could not be performed with batches containing the "normal" or "representative" amount of active substance which normally occurs after validated production runs.

It should also be discussed whether the full range of laboratory tests and field trials have to be performed and which of the tests may be deleted or may be subject to an imposition on a licence. As an alternative to impositions, the use of a conditional licence system could be helpful.

Furthermore, some Ph. Eur. monographs already existing for MUMS vaccines might be revised to facilitate the performance of some tests or to replace or even delete some tests. In parallel, the acceptance of tests not in compliance with Ph. Eur. must be increased, provided the equivalence of an alternative test can be justified. It must be stressed that a pragmatic assessment of this equivalence justification is necessary.

As the revised EU legislation will rely more on risk assessments to evaluate licences, most of the items mentioned can be covered by a Risk/Benefit assessment. But again, a pragmatic approach is necessary.

These are some items for discussion and it would not be surprising if the points presented are regarded as incomplete. The speakers to follow will give their opinion on some of these topics and perhaps on some additional aspects. The goal of this meeting is to provide proposals for a pragmatic reduction of provisions to reach a better availability of IVMPs for MUMS without, however, a reduction in their quality, safety, and efficacy. This sounds like the squaring of the circle but nevertheless efforts should be made in this field to increase the availability of vaccines and to encourage vaccine manufacturers to develop, redevelop and/or re-animate MUMS-IVMPs.

Dr. C. Jungbäck, Paul-Ehrlich-Institut, Paul-Ehrlich-Str. 51-59, D-63225 Langen, Germany.
E-mail: junca@pei.de

Jungbäck C (ed): Consideration of Alternative Licensing Procedures for Vaccines for Minor Species, Minor Indications and Autogenous/Autologous Products.
Dev Biol. Basel, Karger, 2004, vol 117, pp 93-95.

Minor Species, Who Cares?

M.M.L. Aerts

Intervet International BV., Boxmeer, The Netherlands

The main reason why companies do not invest in the development of vaccines for minor species or minor indications is because of the lack of a proper return on the investment required. During the past ten years regulatory requirements on all aspects of the development (Analytical; Safety and Efficacy) have increased. In addition GLP, GMP and GCP regulations have come into force and are becoming stricter every year. Also, the perception of risk and what risk can be accepted has changed significantly towards a situation where the no-risk principle has become predominant in many EU countries. This has led to development times of between six to nine years for vaccines for veterinary use and development costs that have more than doubled during the last 10 years (Fig. 1).

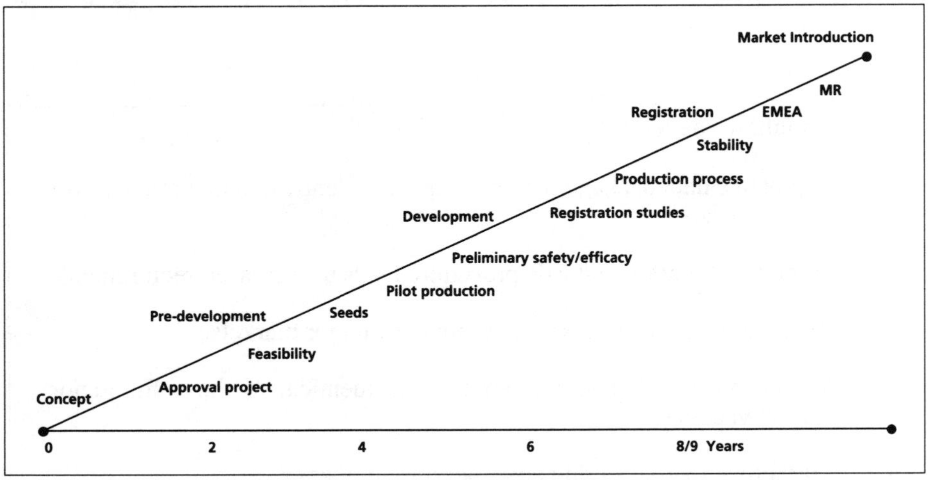

Figure 1.

Market characteristics have not improved, whereas the hurdle for a certain product to enter the market has increased due to the new registration system in the EU. This situation has forced veterinary vaccine companies to put more emphasis on financial criteria when selecting its development projects, whereas innovation and technical feasibility have become relatively less important. The practical consequence is that companies must focus on major markets. Per definition most vaccines for minor species do not present major markets and although (part of) the EU regulatory authorities express their concern that minor species are being neglected, in practice that concern is not reflected in the current registration procedures as used for licensing products intended for application to minor species.

In the current situation, companies cannot respond quickly to emerging diseases, nor are they able to provide vaccines to certain market segments, which are locally or regionally relevant (ducks, rabbits, turkeys, goats). The market itself reacts by an increasing off-label use of existing vaccines, increased use of antibiotics for bacterial diseases and increased use of autogenous vaccines. This approach seems to be opposite to what the EU wants to achieve.

For veterinary vaccine companies there seems to be no incentive for (re) starting development of products for minor markets (Table 1). During the vaccine review process of the past 10 years, many minor market products have disappeared. It is not feasible to produce products economically for only one or two remaining countries because as a consequence of the regulatory environment, a financial loss is the outcome.

Only a thorough and extensive revision of requirements for development, registration and (post-) marketing of vaccines for minor markets will allow vaccine companies to develop products for minor species. This should, and can, be done in a way that allows the development and marketing of vaccines that are safe, efficacious, pure and sterile. Also, a very important step towards facilitating the development and marketing of regulated vaccines would be to simplify the introduction of new strains in existing vaccines with a well-known safety and efficacy profile. Finally, the registration process and the requirements with regard to variations and changes in the Ph. Eur. will also have to be

Table 1.

Why should we develop ?

- ☐ In practice data package for minor species identical to that required for major species
- ☐ Often local market and MR procedure leads to increased requirements
- ☐ Production costs per dose higher than for major markets
- ☐ Maintenance and post-marketing costs identical to those for major market vaccines
- ☐ Marketing and packaging costs per dose higher

critically reviewed and modified. Without such a thorough and extensive revision process only one certainty will remain: very few vaccines for minor markets will be developed and the use of (often non-regulated) autogenous vaccines will increase.

Dr. M.M.L. Aerts, Intervet International BV, Wim de Körverstraat 35, NL-5831 AN Boxmeer, The Netherlands
E-mail: rene.aerts@intervet.com

Jungbäck C (ed): Consideration of Alternative Licensing Procedures for Vaccines for Minor Species, Minor Indications and Autogenous/Autologous Products.
Dev Biol. Basel, Karger, 2004, vol 117, pp 97-103.

Conditional Licensing of Veterinary Biologicals in the United States: a Major Manufacturer's Perspective

M.M. Carlson, Y.-W. Chiang, H.-J. Chu

Fort Dodge Animal Health, Fort Dodge, Iowa, USA

Introduction

Veterinary biologicals are important tools. They have been used for many years to prevent or to reduce the impact of many of the most deadly and costly diseases of animals. In the United States, as in most countries, veterinary vaccines are very heavily regulated. U.S. manufacturers are required to prepare the products under strict government supervision, mandated under the Virus Serum Toxin Act (VSTA) of 1913, as amended in 1985. In passing the VSTA in 1913, Congress assigned to the United States Department of Agriculture (USDA) the authority to ensure veterinary biologicals are not worthless, harmful, dangerous or contaminated. Enforcement of the VSTA remains the responsibility of the USDA Animal and Plant Health Inspection Service (APHIS) Center for Veterinary Biologicals (CVB).

Many detailed rules and guidance documents have been put in force by USDA since the adoption of the VSTA. These regulatory standards constitute a fairly rigid framework inside which U.S. veterinary vaccines must fall.

Estimates vary as to the average time it takes to satisfy the standard USDA licensing requirements for vaccines. For competitive reasons, biologicals manufacturers often closely guard detailed statistics on the subject. At Fort Dodge Animal Health time scales vary, but three to five years to satisfy the USDA biological licensing requirements is not unusual. Many projects involving truly novel technology take much longer.

In ordinary circumstances major manufacturers budget and plan for the satisfaction of the standard USDA requirements as a simple matter of doing business. But in the face of a new disease entity, time periods of three to five years or more are not in the best interest of animals and their owners.

In the VSTA Congress made clear in 1913 and reiterated in 1985 that there should be room made in the regulations for cases where a completely rigid licensing system would be damaging to animal health in the U.S. In the VSTA, Congress allowed USDA to make exceptions to the detailed licensing requirements, particularly during times of disease epidemics. The law contains the following provision: "In order to meet an emergency condition, limited market or local situation, or other special circumstance ...... the Secretary may issue a special license under an expedited procedure on such conditions as are necessary to assure purity, safety, and a reasonable expectation of efficacy."

This expedited procedure provided for in VSTA has become the basis for USDA licensing of autogenous products, regulation of which is described in 9CFR113.113, and for issuance of USDA Conditional Licenses, regulation of which is described in 9CFR 102.6.

What are the Basic Requirements of the Conditional License?

First and foremost, if a fully licensed product is available, a conditional license will not be granted. So the firm must ensure no such product exists, and must be able to demonstrate convincingly that existing products do not, for instance, cross-protect against the agent in question. It is also important to be able to document the real need for the vaccine; does the literature or does documented expert veterinary opinion support the need for the new product? If not, there will be no hope of a conditional license for the vaccine; the licensing company must establish a case that the product is urgently needed, and that it is not in the best interest of animal health in the United States that it be licensed in the ordinary procedure, usually due to the length of time full licensing would be expected to take.

For a product to be eligible for conditional licensing, it must also fall into one (or more) of the three categories approved by Congress: The firm must make a strong argument that the product is needed "in order to meet an emergency condition, limited market or local situation, or other special circumstance."

Emergency conditions have in the past included the identification of new strains of recognized pathogens or altogether new disease entities in the U.S. If a new pathogen is considered by USDA to be a practical candidate for eradication a vaccine to prevent disease caused by that pathogen will not be considered for conditional licensing. Moreover, the mere presence of the organism in the U.S. animal population will not automatically be considered an emergency condition. However, if the organism is causing demonstrable important harm to a significant number of animals, it might be possible for the company to make a case for conditional licensing, arguing that its presence in U.S. animals represents an emergency condition.

Conditional licensing based on the argument that the product is needed to fulfil a need in a limited market or local situation is usually used by companies producing vaccines for use in minor species. Vaccines for pet birds are good examples.

"Local situations" arguments for conditional licensing are rarely used by companies to justify conditional licensing of autogenous products. In theory, where the continuing need for a local autogenous product is established, the conditional licensing procedure would allow commercialization in a wider population of animals and for longer-term use. This avenue is rarely, if ever, actually pursued by autogenous product manufacturers. Instead, autogenous biologicals are frequently used for protracted periods to fulfil local needs.

When companies make a case for conditional licensing, claiming the product is needed due to "special circumstances", the circumstances making full licensing problematic often require extensive documentation. Commonly, this argument is used when the need for the vaccine is well established, the vaccine manufacturing method has been discovered, but at the same time the required experimental challenge model, (for conducting efficacy and/or duration of immunity studies) remains elusive. In this situation, a conditional license can allow the vaccine be made available while the final experiments to prove immunogenicity or duration of immunity conclusively are completed.

If a reasonable case for conditional licensing can be made, then the company must prove purity and safety of the product under the same standards used for full licensing. Full master seed and cell testing is required, and the laboratory and field safety testing requirements are the same as those used for full USDA licensing projects. What is unique for companies pursuing conditional licensing projects is the USDA requirement that the manufacturer prove only a "reasonable expectation" of efficacy. What are considered adequate data to give a "reasonable expectation" are often influenced by the basis on which the argument for licensing was made : If the product is being licensed for a dire emergency, a small study with a serological response might be adequate. If the product is being licensed based on a "special circumstance" argument the protocol for proof of a reasonable expectation of efficacy is often the subject of long negotiation between USDA and the firm, and may involve large field efficacy studies or use of multiple indirect indicators of vaccine effectiveness just short of actual statistically significant differences in clinical disease proved by vaccination/challenge of host animals.

How are Conditionally Licensed Products Different from Autogenous Vaccines ?

The most important difference between Conditionally Licensed Vaccines and Autogenous Vaccines is in the quality specifications and uniformity of production that are required for a conditionally licensed vaccine, but which are not required for autogenous vaccines. Vaccines made under conditional license are made using fully tested master seeds and cells, and under Outlines of Production as detailed as any used for production of fully licensed products. In contrast, autogenous products are not prepared under the master seed concept, and even in those very exceptional instances where an autogenous vaccine strain has been used for an extended period, the conditions of production and testing of the autogenous product originating from the seed is only loosely defined in a general outline of production. The result is that conditionally licensed products typically have important quality advantages in the areas of purity, safety and uniformity of serials when contrasted with autogenous vaccines.

A second area of divergence between conditionally licensed products and autogenous products is that autogenous products both by law and by regulation are made from isolates that arise in a given herd or flock. Autogenous vaccines are intended, under normal circumstances, for use only in this herd or flock of origin. In contrast, conditionally licensed vaccines are intended by the company and by the USDA for broader application to all animals with a need for the product. Conditionally licensed products have no particular link to any single herd or flock. This difference makes application of autogenous vaccines across a veterinarian's practice, outside the originating flock, a complicated bureaucratic exercise. Veterinarians and autogenous producing companies frequently object to the record-keeping burdens related to the herd of origin restrictions.

Use of conditionally licensed vaccines, in contrast, is simple from the vaccine purchaser's perspective, because use of the product is usually only restricted by state or region, and not user-by-user. State-wide restrictions are handled for the most part, by the manufacturer.

Many veterinarians and most animal owners do not understand the difference between autogenous vaccines and conditionally licensed vaccines. Even very well informed academicians are not aware of the fundamental differences, and call for liberalization of autogenous rules. In many cases purchasers of autogenous products do not realize the different standard for purity and safety implicit in the nature of those products, and often users' past experience with autogenous vaccines leads to unwarranted concern about the use of conditional licensed products due to the confusion of the two product standards.

How is a Conditional License Different from a "Full" USDA License?

The difference between demonstrating efficacy and demonstrating a reasonable expectation of efficacy is the primary difference for the company as it pursues either full or conditional USDA licensing plans. As mentioned earlier, this difference can be greater or lesser depending on the product and the state of the science related to the disease. A second important difference can be in the potency test requirement, which without a final efficacy demonstration is usually not completely validated. All conditionally licensed products must be tested for potency, but frequently the test is preliminary in nature and must be updated before attaining a full license.

Fully licensed products in the United States are usually freely sold across the United States, and most fully licensed products are legally sold to veterinarians and non-veterinarians alike. Conditionally licensed vaccines, in contrast, are often restricted to sales to veterinarians only and always require approval from each of the 50 states' official state veterinarians. Each state can further impose special restrictions and reporting requirements for his area of authority. This is an important consideration for large companies, as the paperwork burden can be substantial. When selling conditionally licensed products, excellent computerized inventory and distribution controls and an unimpeachable audit trail are essential to large companies in order to manage the complex record-keeping and reporting functions across 50 states.

USDA and/or the state authorities may also impose other special restrictions on conditionally licensed products. Examples include special pharmaco-vigilance requirements and requirements for pre-approval of advertising and promotional materials. In some unusual circumstances, states can require pre-approval of individual customers as recipients based on state permit procedures. Some states create consumer notification requirements which must be fulfilled by the companies. Conditional licenses are issued for only a limited time set by the USDA. The manufacturer must report progress made toward satisfying full license requirements on a regular (usually annual) basis. If the manufacturer fails to defend the track record of progress, USDA can permit the product license to be terminated.

Can Conditional Licenses be Converted to "Full" USDA Licenses?

Some conditionally licensed vaccines never progress to the point where they become standard vaccines in the veterinarian's basic toolkit. But in some famous cases conditional licensing served as the first big step made by manufacturers in introducing important novel products into the U.S. market. A short list of examples of former conditionally licensed vaccines now available as fully licensed products includes PRRS vaccine (Boehringer Ingelheim), SIV serotype H3N2 vaccine (Schering Plough Animal Health), Borrelia burgdorferi bacterin (FDAH). In some cases the manufacturer used the conditional license period to collect important field efficacy data, thus helping to resolve some final questions in favour of the product.

What are the Essential Considerations for a Manufacturer in Preparing to Market a Vaccine under Conditional License?

A practical fact of life in our industry is that conditionally licensed vaccines cannot compete favorably with fully licensed vaccines, due to consumer confidence being greater (understandably) in fully licensed vaccines. So companies try to be first in conditional licensing, hoping their conditional license can then be rapidly converted to a full license. For small companies the income from sale of the conditionally licensed vaccine can fund the completion of the efficacy studies needed for full licensing.

Large firms such as FDAH tend to concentrate any conditional license activities in the major species where the return on investment in vaccines is seen as greater, while small companies with more concentration in niche markets are more likely to pursue minor species products successfully. Several companies, both large and small, have made important vaccines available for the first time in the United States using the conditional licensing procedure. An important consideration is whether the extensive record-keeping and reporting burden that comes with conditional licensing is worthwhile for the company.

Two Case Studies from FDAH

Equine Rotavirus Vaccine was conditionally licensed by Fort Dodge Animal Health on January 3, 1996, and remains conditionally licensed today. The demand for this vaccine originated in Kentucky, where scientists at the Gluck Center had reported foal losses due to rotavirus-associated diarrhoea could be reduced by use of a novel vaccine.

The need for a vaccine was clear, on at least a regional basis, and the region was the most important equine region of the United States. Commercial development of the vaccine was challenging, but FDAH scientists working with the Gluck Center came up with a vaccine that generated good antibody responses. The vaccine also showed good field study performance. Proof of efficacy using standard host animal vaccination challenge techniques proved a major stumbling block, however, due to the lack of a satisfactory challenge model. FDAH appealed for conditional licensing of the vaccine based on an argument that the lack of a challenge model was a special circumstance.

Since conditional licensing, FDAH has worked to conduct field and laboratory efficacy studies. These studies have so far not completely satisfied USDA requirements for full licensing. In the meantime, however, the Gluck Center scientists continue to support the importance of this vaccine for mares in Kentucky. From an FDAH perspective, this product has become a rather regionally important product and Kentuckians strongly support the conditional license re-issue each year.

West Nile Virus Vaccine was conditionally licensed based on FDAH's appeal that an emergency situation had developed which had led to an urgent need for the vaccine in the United States in the summer of 2001. This vaccine licensing project began in 1999, when equine and medical cases of WNV encephalitis were first diagnosed in the United States. By the time the virus appeared in the form of a full-blown outbreak of mosquito-borne encephalitis in northwestern Florida in late July 2001, FDAH had completed full master seed and cell testing, vaccine formulation studies, and large host animal serological response studies. The production and testing specifications had also been set and consistency batches had been made. A full-scale field safety test in horses in several eastern U.S. states had been done. When Florida officials reported the urgent need for vaccine to contain serious equine losses in that state, USDA responded by issuing the conditional license for the FDAH vaccine. The WNV virus spread during the summer and autumn of 2001 across the eastern half of the U.S. and is now present in 47 of the lower 48 states.

There were many questions and concerns in 2000 about the use of a conditionally licensed product in very valuable horses, especially in areas of the U.S. which were not considered to be in the direct path of the virus. The confusion on the part of the public concerning how conditional and fully licensed products differed contributed to the concern. But the impact of vaccination on losses due to the disease was felt almost immediately. And the rapid movement of the virus in the completely naïve U.S. environment made vaccination more and more important.

The full license for the WNV product was issued on February 6, 2003, when FDAH had satisfied USDA requirements for vaccination/challenge and duration of immunity studies and had completed validation of the potency test in line with those studies. The quality of the conditionally licensed WNV vaccine was supported by its ultimately satisfying full USDA licensing requirements.

Use of this vaccine during the 18 months it was conditionally licensed is credited with saving the lives of many thousands of horses that might otherwise have died of West Nile Viral Encephalitis. In retrospect, the wisdom of the authors of the VSTA in providing for the expedited conditional license procedure is clear.

Conclusions

1. Conditional licensing is a procedure that allows manufacturing companies to respond rapidly and effectively during exceptional times, in the best interests of animals and their owners.
2. The procedure gives rapid widespread product availability, and assures uniform quality.
3. The conditional licensing procedure fosters and rewards innovation while protecting the public interest.

Dr. M.M. Carlson, U.S. and Canada Biological Regulatory Affairs, Fort Dodge Animal Health, 800 Fifth Street N.W., P.O. Box 518, Fort Dodge, Iowa 50501, USA.
E-mail: mcarlson@fdah.com

Jungbäck C (ed): Consideration of Alternative Licensing Procedures for Vaccines for Minor Species, Minor Indications and Autogenous/Autologous Products.
Dev Biol. Basel, Karger, 2004, vol 117, pp 105-110.

Vaccines for Minor Use and Minor Species (MUMS) – Industry's Views

B. Bönisch

Merial S.A.S., Lyon, France

Abstract: Over the past 30 years the importance of vaccines for minor use and minor species has changed for multinational animal health companies. The major reasons for this are being reviewed, with a particular focus on technical, financial and business aspects. Key regulatory obstacles to the development of new products for minor uses and minor species are identified, and examples of vaccines falling into the various categories are provided. A number of proposals are offered with the intention of resolving the medicines availability problem between all the stakeholders involved. Finally, based on the presented scientific and regulatory considerations, ideas are shared as to where the legal and economical framework would need to change to reach a viable solution.

INTRODUCTION

The views presented in this paper reflect the European perspective. Examples of MUMS vaccines as well as reflections on possible problem resolutions given later on in the text should be seen in this context.

The development focus of the company was originally on vaccines for major food-producing animal and companion animal species, with a specific emphasis on diseases of major health impact. Then, in France during the 1970s, intensive breeding and rearing of rabbits and ducks started. This new management of animal production led to serious health problems related with a high mortality. At the origin were diseases such as myxomatosis or parvovirosis. In an attempt to find solutions to the problems rapidly, coalitions were formed between breeders, industry and government laboratories with the shared objective of identifying remedies, which could be available quickly, while at the same time maintaining an acceptable level of product safety and efficacy.

In the early 1980s, many companies became international, then global. This resulted in the establishment of business operations in countries within Europe and throughout the world. With the subsequent change of the market from a purely national size to global dimensions, automatically a previously important minor species market such as France became less significant relative to the overall global market potential for the company.

A third major evolution affecting all animal health companies was the increase of regulatory requirements, particularly throughout the 1990s. This resulted in much higher R & D expenses and a prolongation in the time to market for new products. Out of the necessity to recuperate R & D investments, companies had to focus their R & D resources on the development and maintenance of products for major species, diseases and markets. Directly linked to these increased regulatory requirements, the business interest to invest in MUMS vaccines for species such as ducks, rabbits, pigeons, goats, cage and game birds declined.

The situation was further aggravated due to the loss of MUMS products as a consequence of the review of veterinary vaccines, applying new regulatory requirements to existing products. Often, to retain the approved MUMS vaccines, firms would need to conduct additional experimental work, to upgrade registration dossiers in line with current requirements. For a number of products, in view of the limited market size and the limited potential return on investment, companies had to make the decision not to invest in a renewal of the marketing authorisation and to withdraw the product from the market.

Scientific and Technical Considerations

In the following a number of scientific and technical observations will be reviewed, several of which would be useful to consider in the process of finding a solution to the medicines availability problem since they mitigate the high standard regulations.

A number of previously important diseases became less so over time, due to improved management practices or a decrease in prevalence through control (eradication) programmes. As a result, companies are no longer involved in these market segments, a circumstance which has had a negative impact on minor species.

Numerous new pathogens were identified during the past two decades, often afflicting minor species. Today's diseases frequently present with a clinical profile that is less definitive than the major epidemics of past decades and frequently manifesting reduced production performance instead of high morbidity and mortality. As a result, the demonstration of vaccine efficacy against the causal pathogen tends to be less straightforward than was the case with the old, classical diseases.

Technical difficulties are being faced in obtaining SPF or maternal antibody-free animals of certain minor species, an aspect which would need to be considered in the regulation of products to treat these species.

For existing products with limited or no efficacy data in conformity with current regulatory requirements, disease outbreaks are reported in markets where these licensed vaccines are no longer available. These observations indicate the probable efficacy of such products in the absence of the data required to support the new registration requirements.

The same pathogen may cause a disease in different species, e.g. haemorrhagic enteritis in turkeys and marble spleen disease in pheasants caused by adenovirus, paratuberculosis and chlamydiosis in ruminants, pneumovirosis and pasteurellosis in chicken, turkey and duck as well as clostridiosis in ruminants and pigs.

A differentiation can be made between live and inactivated vaccines as well as between diseases of purely economic importance (e.g. decreased production performance) and diseases posing a true animal welfare or safety concern (e.g. high mortality, zoonoses).

Moreover, different conditions are being faced during field use of a product than during regulatory trials. Thus infield management standards often vary, the number of animals treated with a given product is many times higher, and the use of vaccine may not always be in line with the recommended dosage regimen. In addition, challenges conducted during product development are often more severe than those faced in the field. Finally, wide field use of a product usually leads to rapid identification of problem cases (e.g. within two weeks in the poultry industry).

Financial Obstacles

There are a number of financial obstacles which have a negative impact on the availability of MUMS products. The cost related to the use of vaccines is related to the amount of meat produced from the treated animal rather than to the number of heads treated.

As a result of the globalisation of the animal health industry, the economic importance of a minor species to a country, which may be important from a local or national perspective, often loses significance from the perspective of a multinational company that requires a reasonable return on product development investment.

In the case of a MUMS product the required selling price is frequently incompatible with the economic realities of the target market.

Last but not least affecting the incentive for firms to license vaccines for MUMS are the costs involved with product maintenance (i.e. generation of new data for renewals, variations, fees, changes of packaging) and manufacturing (including the cost of goods for country-specific packaging). These regulatory requirements present a significant burden to maintaining existing products on the market and are factored into the return on investment considerations for launching new ones.

Regulatory Barriers to New Vaccine Development

While 30 years ago all stakeholders involved in MUMS vaccine development and registration mainly aimed at rapidly finding a solution to major health problems, the focus today has shifted to optimising production performance and the avoidance of any risk linked to product use. This development clearly is not advantageous for MUMS products.

The existing system for "provisional authorisation" of products has proved to be extremely resource-intensive for industry. Licences need to be renewed annually and a full-blown product development conducted and submitted to the competent authorities to transfer the licence into a full marketing authorisation. While this is a useful concept for major species and indication products, it is not seen as a viable option for MUMS products. The high R & D costs, fees, and the amount of regulatory work required for maintenance of provisional licences result in a negative cost/benefit ratio for industry.

New regulatory requirements are being applied to existing products possessing a long history of proven safety and efficacy under in-field-use conditions. This practice has led to the removal of approved products from the market, further aggravating the availability of products for MUMS.

Examples

Examples of vaccines used for minor species: myxomatosis in the rabbit, parvovirosis in the duck, haemorrhagic enteritis in the turkey, canary pox in canaries, salmonella vaccine in pigeons and paramyxovirus/pigeon pox virus in pigeons.

Vaccines for minor use comprise paratuberculosis for ruminants, rabies in cattle, sheep, horses and other rabies-sensitive species, as well as tetanus in cattle, sheep, pigs, dogs, cats and other tetanus-sensitive species. Equine rota virus for pregnant mares, equine arteritis virus for stallions, rabies in ferrets and distemper in ferrets would be examples of vaccines for minor species and minor uses. Looking for examples of vaccines which are lacking for minor species and minor uses, contagious agalactia in goats, caprine arthritis and encephalitis in goats, salmonella abortus ovis and border disease in sheep qualify for this category.

It is also known from the field that major products are being used off-label, a practice which cannot be supported or recommended by the marketing authorisation holder. Examples of such off-label use are products for broiler chickens which are being used in layers and breeders, products for cattle or sheep administered to goats and products for chickens used in turkeys, ducks and game birds (e.g. in the case of Marek's, EDS, influenza vaccine for turkeys, IB vaccine for pheasants). Moreover, in the field, routes of administration different from those on the label are being used.

Ways to Satisfy the Product Needs for Minor Species/Minor Uses

In view of the many obstacles impeding the development and maintenance of MUMS products, it will be essential that efforts in this area concentrate on the most important pathogens. Assurance that these are properly identified could be obtained by close collaboration between users in need of a solution to a health problem, epidemiological centres, and industry. The objectivity of the decision-making process could be guaranteed by an independent body such as the EU Commission.

Clearly the financial obstacles preventing manufacturers from developing and producing MUMS vaccines would need to be addressed and ways identified to obtain subsidies to support the timely provision of urgently needed products. Another incentive for industry to invest in developing and maintaining MUMS vaccines would be the relaxation of regulatory requirements to the degree this is possible in a given situation without compromising in an irresponsible manner the quality, safety and efficacy of the specific product in question. Among the possible changes which could be considered in the context of the EU regulatory framework are the following:

A more pragmatic approach towards the evaluation of the quality, safety and efficacy of MUMS products that balances the potential risks and benefits of the product, coupled with due consideration given to the impact and importance of the specific disease/pathogen. Diseases having animal welfare and human health concerns would be evaluated differently from diseases solely affecting productivity performance. Likewise, existing products for which field experience and pharmacovigilance data are available would be evaluated differently from new product developments. A product already available for other species or indications will take an intermediate position between the above two scenarios. Consideration should be evaluated relative to the use of extrapolation or data and experience from one species or sub-population to another (e.g. on the basis of the causal pathogen or the field experience from off-label use).

It would be preferable to have one single European body (i.e. the Committee for Veterinary Medicinal Products, CVMP) in charge of the assessment and evaluation of the various cases potentially qualifying for a pragmatic MUMS approach to ensure consistency in decision-making throughout the EU.

A further point not to be neglected is the necessity not only to reduce current quality, safety and efficacy requirements, but also certain procedural aspects of the registration process which today render the system burdensome and costly. A refinement of labelling requirements, allowing for less information on the label, as compared to that required for fully developed products, would be consistent with requirements for packaging literature to reflect the actual data package available and assessed for MUMS product approval (e.g. limited information on efficacy). Additionally, less text on the label would permit multi-language packaging and decrease the need for country-specific packs, thus reducing the cost of goods. Also the possibility of fee waivers for both first marketing authorisation application as well as subsequent variations should be considered. Overall, a reduction of the administrative requirements would need to be attempted and the detailed possibilities for action in that area investigated.

Conclusions

All parties affected by the limited availability of products for MUMS today are fully aware of the issue. Subsequent to the first major conference organised on Medicines Availability (Brussels, July 1999), major contributions towards problem resolution have been made by the EU Commission, the European Agency for the Evaluation of Medicinal Products, the CVMP and other stakeholders. In particular, the CVMP is to be commended on the recent elaboration of a position paper resulting in a number of proposals to address the problem. This document has been distributed for consultation and once finalised, it will become a fundamental platform from which further actions will evolve in the resolution of the current product gap for MUMS. It is important to use occasions like this current conference to define viable future legal and economic frameworks supporting MUMS products further.

A major pre-requisite for problem resolution is the preparedness by all parties to accept products which may have certain gaps and to share the risks involved. The extent of the regulatory data package supporting a MUMS product should be a function of the scientific evidence available to support the specific case and of the resulting risk/benefit ratio. Finally, the need to overcome the financial obstacles will need to be addressed.

Acknowledgements

The author would like to acknowledge the contribution of a number of colleagues without whose help compilation of the information presented would not have been possible, i.e. Daniel Gaudry, Jacques Léchenet, Peter Cargill, Jean-Marc Lalloz, Bernard-Fernand Devaux and Norman Habermehl.

Dr. B. Bönisch, Merial S.A.S., 29, avenue Tony Garnier, F-69348 Lyon Cedex 07, France.
E-mail: brigitte.boenisch@merial.com

Jungbäck C (ed): Consideration of Alternative Licensing Procedures for Vaccines for Minor Species, Minor Indications and Autogenous/Autologous Products.
Dev Biol. Basel, Karger, 2004, vol 117, pp 111-116.

A Small Manufacturer's Perspective on Small Volume Products

J.N. Huff

Colorado Serum Company, Denver, CO, USA

I would like to share with you the experiences our company, Colorado Serum Company, has had with licensing procedures for Minor Use/Minor Species products; what we see as the positive and negative aspects of Conditional Licences, and then suggest improvements to the licensing system to meet what we see as current day needs.

Colorado Serum Company is a privately owned firm located in Denver, Colorado. My grandfather, a veterinarian, founded the company in 1923 to manufacture Hog Cholera Antiserum. Today we produce about 35 veterinary biologicals – vaccines, bacterins, and antisera – and a line of veterinary instruments, all primarily for use in large animals. We employ about 100 people and our facilities occupy 22 acres within the city of Denver. We distribute our products throughout the world. Nevertheless, by U.S. standards we are still considered to be a "small manufacturer."

When Colorado Serum Company considers Minor Use/Minor Species products, we look to the USDA framework of "Conditional License." In the recent past we have had experience with Conditionally Licensing at least five different products and we have three current projects which we believe are candidates for a Conditional License.

The five Conditional Licenses have covered a wide variety of types of products and have resulted in a wide variety of outcomes. Our experiences of these five products are:

1. Ram Epididymitis Bacterin (Brucella Ovis)

This product certainly qualifies as a Minor Use/Minor Species since sheep in the U.S. are often considered a Minor Species and breeding rams even more so. We made this product specifically at the request of the Colorado Woolgrowers and originally it was only used in the State of Colorado. After completing the requirements for a full regular licence, it was sold extensively throughout the U.S. Today, because of test and culling programs, the usage is extremely small; however we continue to make it available.

2. Ovine Chlamydia Psittaci Bacterin

Even though sheep numbers are considered minor, Chlamydia abortions are a major problem. We obtained a Conditional License for this product while efficacy testing was underway, which also provided for widespread field safety data. The requirement to obtain 50 state approvals became very burdensome, resulting in too many modes of use and distribution. Some states had no restrictions, and others, for example, restricted the use only to Veterinarians. Coupled with the fact that the product was sold by many interstate distributors, the plan became unworkable. Fortunately, very soon the product was fully licensed and also used in combinations, and continues today to be an important product, both to sheep producers and ourselves.

3. Vesicular Stomatitis Vaccine

Responding to an emergency outbreak situation in the U.S. several years ago, our company as well as others, quickly received a Conditional License for a killed vaccine. In spite of the rapid response of both the USDA and manufacturers, the product was never widely used when it first became available, and within a year the outbreak seemed to disappear naturally, and with it the demand. The Conditional Licenses were not renewed, and no manufacturer had any desire to follow-up with any further licensing work. We were left with a very large inventory, which we had to dispose of, and we had to adsorb all the costs.

4. Brucella Abortus Vaccine, RB-51

This is probably our best success story. This product certainly does not fit the Minor Use/Minor Species definition; however, because of the U.S. Brucellosis Eradication Program, it was an excellent candidate for a Conditional License. The rapid availability of this product allowed the programme to proceed quickly because vaccination did not interfere with disease testing, and it allowed the federal government to maintain control over use, distribution, and record-keeping. The efficacy testing requirements and Environmental Impact Statement presented so many difficulties that only the close cooperation between our company and the USDA could have resulted in any licensing of the product. Today the product has a full regular licence.

5. Caprine Serum Fraction – Immunomodulator

This product has certainly been one of the most unique experiences we have ever had. It definitely qualifies as a Minor Use/Minor Species product. It is an adjunct therapy for use primarily in athletic horses to reduce recovery time from lower respiratory disease significantly. Considerable field efficacy testing demonstrated that the product has a significant effect and that it was safe, but the biological mode of action could not be shown. It took us about five years to obtain a Conditional License pending development of a potency test. These efforts were continually unsuccessful due to the lack of understanding of the biological activity. We maintained that only a chemistry type of potency test could be developed; however USDA required us to continue to explore all avenues to develop a biological activity test for an additional five years, until we all gave up and the products obtained a full regular licence.

All these experiences have given us the opportunity to develop some very clear feelings and opinions about the USDA Conditional License framework, so I should now like to explain what we see as the positives, negatives, and the really negatives about Conditional Licenses, or what I call the Good, the Bad, and the Ugly.

The Good

There are certainly many aspects of Conditional Licenses that are good for animal owners, manufacturers, and even regulatory bodies. This approach can lead to a much quicker time to market, which benefits the animal owner, the manufacturer, and even provides good public relations for the USDA. By allowing for products with "conditional" label recommendations, there can be a reduction in "off-label" use of products, which could be more likely to result in untoward outcomes, both in safety and efficacy. Conditional Licensing provides a high level and comfort of product manufacturing and distribution control that is not present when such products might be made illegally. In other words, any level of licensing is better than none at all.

The Bad

There are, however, inherent aspects to Conditional Licenses that make this avenue more difficult than perhaps it should be. In spite of the shorter time to licensing, Conditional Licensing is still not what some might consider "fast-track". All the same bureaucratic obstacles and limitations exist for Conditional Licenses as for a Full Regular License. The criteria USDA use for Conditional Licenses are sometime still very difficult to define, and these criteria are described in very subjective terms. Definitions such as "satisfactory progress", "may", and "reasonable" are open to many interpretations. Even "minor use" and "minor species" are hard to quantify. We feel that the expectation that all Conditional Licenses will result in a full regular licence is sometimes unrealistic. There is, in our opinion, a place for products that might never be able to rise to the proof of efficacy requirements of a full regular licence.

The Ugly

Finally, there are several issues that we feel thwart the intent of the Conditional License scheme. The requirement for one-year renewals creates an additional demand for paperwork application, review times, and sidetracks efforts toward the important goal. In our experience, rarely can much be accomplished in a year. Additionally, the six-month limitation on other manufacturers after issue of one full regular licence raises all sorts of competitive problems. Label restrictions, such as no use of trade names and advertising reviews, serve no purpose, in our opinion. There obviously are certain products that by their nature might be restricted to certain States or geographical areas, but for most products, the requirement for individual State permission is burdensome and unreasonable. In most instances, I believe that if a product is good enough to be Conditionally Licensed, it is good enough to be used anywhere.

Nevertheless, in spite of what might seem a negative view, our firm sees great value in the concept of Conditional Licenses, yet when we look at the spectrum of requirements for different types of licences it seems that things are clustered at either end with not much in the middle. Autogenous products meet rigid manufacturing standards; however there is never any requirement for proof of field efficacy or host safety. Conditional Licenses must start with a high level of field safety and a "reasonable expectation of efficacy", and then move briskly and inevitably toward a full licence.

It appears to us that in today's world there are circumstances that call for special licences for special products, including Minor Use/Minor Species, which fall between these extremes. There are five special circumstances that seem to justify special products: financial, time, regulatory, technical, and social.

(i) Financial

One of the greatest obstacles to development of any biological product is the financial resources necessary not only to complete licensing requirements, but even to perform the necessary research and development to bring forward a potential product. In addition there are financial obligations for continuing support of a full regular licence. Most companies can reasonably justify this commitment if the potential payback is worthwhile. This is simply not the case with Minor Use/Minor Species. Secondarily, we find that many large companies have no interest in limited market products regardless of any special licensing accommodations.

(ii) Time

Not only are there many instances where the immediate availability of a product is crucial to animal health, but also, as the old saying goes, "time is money" and time becomes a financial issue.

(iii) Regulatory

There are instances where diseases have very widespread geographical implications, for example, when they may adversely affect imports or exports. In these cases, it could be in the national interest of a country to have the availability of a biological product. Even more so, in the case of animal health emergencies, product availability can greatly enhance and speed conclusions. And perhaps most importantly, if a licensed product is not available, there is always the prospect of illegally imported products, dangerous off-label usage, and uncontrolled private manufacturing.

(iv) Technical

Unfortunately what we often have to deal with today is what I term "difficult diseases". These are ones that sometimes cannot be successfully or repeatedly reproduced, or those that only cause animals to be non-viable, if not sick. Perhaps worst of all, there still remain many animal diseases which are serious human pathogens. Not only is there reluctance on the part of many companies to even work with these, but also classic vaccination/challenge tests can be dangerous to humans if not unnecessarily inhumane to animals. Also, there are many fully licensed products already available that could have expanded label claims for Minor Use/Minor Species. Currently it is our understanding that it is not possible for a product to be both fully and conditionally licensed.

(v) Social

Finally there are social issues and political pressures that go far beyond the scientific arena. There are emerging animal industries, at least in the U.S., that involve what have previously been considered minor species. There are scientific and social pressures to reduce the use of antibiotics in animals and humans, and biologicals may offer the best hope of replacement. Animal welfare concerns are driving more decisions concerning animal testing and product usage. And in today's culture, there is a wide spectrum of human values. Gone are the days where, frankly speaking, most consumers trust governments to make decisions for them. They want more information and the empowerment of choices, right or wrong. We see widely disparate views among animal owners and even veterinarians concerning the levels of safety and efficacy they expect from a licensed product. There are different kinds of people and they want different kinds of products.

After this consideration of the advantages and disadvantages of the current position, including the concerns and needs of animal owners, veterinarians, and manufacturers, what is the prescription for the prescription?

First, matters which are unlikely to succeed and which do not provide long-term solutions.

Poor Solutions

I have looked at the proposed U.S. FDA style of Minor Use/Minor Species legislation, and it does not seem to address problems in a satisfactory manner. Firstly, it is not usable for food-producing animals, and while it does provide some relief, it does not go far enough. Secondly, except in extreme cases, I am philosophically opposed to programmes that depend upon government funding or grants. In our experiences there is always far too much attached to it. We are looking for reductions in paperwork, costs, and time, and no government programme seems to do that. However, perhaps the worst solution is to not provide for these types of products at all.

So, what might work? I believe it must all start with a philosophical paradigm shift. I would like to suggest that use and need of biologicals – whether Minor Use/Minor Species or not – and in fact of any product, is all about perceived value. A product could be perfectly safe and absolutely efficacious, and yet never used if it does not address a relevant problem or is too expensive. And vice-versa: a product of questionable safety or efficacy could be in great demand if the user feels it adds "value".

I am suggesting that the paradigm shift is all about relative values. In the U.S., I have seen over the last several decades a slow but steady direction on the part of the USDA to move toward higher quality products and stricter licensing requirements.

This is best reflected in the 1985 Amendments to the Virus-Serum-Toxin Act that spelled out that by regulation products must be pure, safe, potent, and efficacious. But these terms can become moving targets and it is, I believe, the nature of government regulatory agencies always to move them higher. This is distinctly different from the original language of the Act that mandated no product could be worthless, dangerous, contaminated or harmful.

I would like to suggest that "perceived value" lies between these two factors and that, in fact, it is situated differently for different people. I believe there is a need for a Special License format to address this in-between area. This would have a two-fold purpose:

- Firstly, do no harm. It would be a disservice, if not a disaster, not to assure safety and purity of any product, and yet that is what can happen if there is no legal provision for product availability.
- Secondly, such products will provide consumers with a choice and availability of treatments. It can also provide important field data that in most instances can be very valuable.

On a more specific level, we would like to see the following elements of such a special licence. On the same level as a full regular licence should be manufacturing controls such as master seed requirements and ingredients sourcing and quality control items such as sterility, safety testing, and record-keeping. Complete available product information and vaccino-vigilance should be the same. However, the special circumstances for special products can be accommodated by greatly reduced or flexible requirements for potency and efficacy. Replacing the term "reasonable expectation of efficacy" with "undetermined" would certainly be more flexible. I believe there needs to be a recognition that some products may never make their way to a full regular licence, and this would be acceptable. It should also be acceptable if one manufacturer pushes their product to full licence and another does not. In most instances such products should not be limited to distribution restrictions. This is a bureaucratic nightmare and virtually impossible to police. Moreover, labelling restrictions must have a practical application. Additionally, review times need to be as short as possible.

So, in conclusion, my assessment is that:

We need to look at a wider picture than just Minor Use/Minor Species. We certainly need to consider licensing alternatives for Minor Use/Minor Species, but this should be part of a larger consideration of alternative licences for many types of product.

We need to work to find ways to make products available and keep products available – to give consumers choices.

At the same time we must not compromise security and safety.

Dr. J.N. Huff, Colorado Serum Company, 4950 York St., Denver, CO 80216, USA.
E-mail: joehuff@colorado-serum.com

Jungbäck C (ed): Consideration of Alternative Licensing Procedures for Vaccines for Minor Species, Minor Indications and Autogenous/Autologous Products.
Dev Biol. Basel, Karger, 2004, vol 117, pp 117-121.

Consideration of Alternative Licensing Procedures for Vaccines for Minor Species and Minor Indications – Manufacturers' Point of View

J. de Foucauld

Ceva-Phylaxia, Budapest, Hungary

Abstract: The E.U. authorities, manufacturers and people in the field are well aware of the need for a smoother, less-demanding and more harmonised way of granting marketing authorisations for certain products.
The authorities have already made some good proposals and this is a basis for discussion and moving ahead. In addition, most of the actors concerned in this process have already had some good (and bad) experiences on how the current system works (or not) in delivering timely authorisations to answer needs from the field, and this factor will also help.
It must be noted that the set goal is quite ambitious. Once an agreement is reached on modified technical and regulatory requirements, it could be requested that both E.U. and national law/guidelines be modified. Clearly this will be a very long process.
Ceva's paper focuses on what could be the best use of current E.U. law for the registration of Minor Species and Minor Indications vaccines. Furthermore, based on first-hand experience, we will detail how the law could be applied in practical ways so that most of the needs are answered as soon as possible and with reasonable data package and registration procedures.

Introduction

The E.U. law for the registration of veterinary biologicals as it developed through the years is clearly aiming at three goals: Safety, Quality and Efficacy, the first being considered above the others concerning the health of the consumers, and the health of the vaccinated animals.

Now that the law has been largely implemented, it appears that many species or indications have been left aside (marketing authorisations abandoned, on hold…) by manufacturers, for lack of means, time, or because "MUMS" were no longer a part of their strategic goals.

This is a result we could expect, since the cost of the requirements was not taken into account when setting the registration system. In many instances there is no difference between the human and veterinary technical requirements but the difference in size between both markets is obvious, even without mentioning vaccines for "MUMS".

The fact that E.U. markets have lost many prevention tools these last years has alerted the E.U. registration authorities, who themselves realised the excessive side of the "system" for these kinds of products, although at the same time, the E.U. commission is largely preoccupied by human health issues and to a lesser extent by the threat of large epizootic diseases. It seems that "MUMS" issues are high on the E.U. political agenda only when at least one of these two conditions is met. Therefore, any goal aiming at changing the law and requirements, in order to bring more flexibility to the registration system, is very ambitious, even if the main actors are pushing for it; furthermore, the process will take considerable time.

Meanwhile, Ceva believes that we can use the current legislative environment to make some rapid progresses in the registration of "MUMS" vaccines. Using the past experiences of the interpretation of the law by different member states and some assessment tools, authorities – with the help of the customers and manufacturers – would be able to grant the needed marketing authorisations.

How Can we Apply the Current E.U. Law: Practical Situations and Proposals

The legal basis from which all actions can be put in place can be found in E.U. Directive 2001/82EC (Official Journal of the European Communities – 28 November 2001). Five articles are involved to some extent and we believe that these articles of the law give considerable flexibility but it requires a great sense of responsibility from both sides – authorities and manufacturers.

We will explain in detail what these articles say, how they are implemented and make some proposals on how to apply them in a more practical way.

Article 4-second paragraph of E.U. Directive 2001/82EC states:

Member States may permit exemptions on their territory in respect of veterinary medicinal products intended solely for aquarium fish, cage birds, homing pigeons, terrarium animals and small rodents, from the provisions in Articles 5, 7 and 8, provided that such products do not contain substances the use of which requires veterinary control and that all possible measures have been taken to prevent unauthorised use of the products for other animals.

This article shows that E.U. authorities had initially planned special provisions in the law for some very minor species. It applies especially to vaccines where there are no MRL issues. It is obvious also that inactivated vaccines are the best candidates in this case, although some precautions must be taken in order to prevent the misuse of the then authorised vaccines. Unfortunately, it appears that very few authorities have implemented this article and that the full registration process is required for vaccines intended for these species.

What should the registration dossier contain? The law clearly states that the applicant is exempted from the provisions of article 5 which requests the full technical and administrative process as stated later in the directive. Therefore authorities and the manufacturer should agree on a minimum content, based on the nature of the vaccine, the target species and the disease involved. Subsequently, based on repeated experiences across the EU, a kind of practical guideline could emerge although all the processes would stay purely at the national level. It is quite certain that the markets for these vaccines will not allow for the heavy, administrative and technical registration work required by the mutual recognition procedure.

Article 7 of E.U. Directive 81/852 states:

Where the health situation so requires, a Member State may authorise the marketing or administration to animals of veterinary medicinal products, which have been authorised by another Member State in accordance with this Directive.

We believe that this is probably the most important article of the E.U. law serving the purpose of "MUMS". Under its provisions, Member States can grant a marketing authorisation (MA) without any lengthy registration procedure. Although some authorities in the E.U. implement this article, it seems that the E.U. commission is reluctant to accept its wide use.

To address the issue, we need to find a good rationale for its application. The justification of the needs should be based, as requested, on the health situation in the target species. Epidemiology and (when relevant) zoonotic aspects, should be detailed along with the economical and possible social consequences from the lack of available product.

Furthermore, the manufacturer should provide the authorities with the "EU Directive 2001/82EC-level" approved SPC from any other Member State and when needed a pharmaco-vigilance follow-up report (PSUR) from the country where the vaccine is already used. If applied, this article would be the groundwork for marketing authorisations based on the 'real' mutual recognition.

Manufacturers can be ready to register a minor-use or minor-species vaccine in the country that first requested it or where the market is bigger (in relative terms), although most manufacturers will not be able to defend the same vaccine through MRP. Even if there is an agreement on a reasonable data package for "MUMS" registration dossiers, in some instances the administrative difficulties through the process or quite simply cost, will bar them from trying. As said earlier, the E.U. system is just not geared for small products! In conclusion, this directive article gives a good occasion to put into practice the flexibility needed and at the same time following the spirit of the E.U. registration system.

Article 8 of E.U. Directive 2001/82EC states:

In the event of serious disease epidemic, Member States may provisionally allow the use of immunological veterinary medicinal products without an authorisation for placing on the market, in the absence of a suitable medicinal product and after informing the Commission of the detailed conditions of use.

In this article Member States have a very strong autonomous power to give an authorisation for temporary use of a vaccine never registered in the E.U. Restrictions are obvious in the article: serious epizootic and provisional authorisation. It is applied on some occasions in the countries that have introduced this article in their national law.

The prerequisites for an Authorisation for Temporary Use (or ATU) are:

- Serious epidemics: (not always easy to judge). For minor species/use, serious can mean small at the national level, although it could be a serious problem for the farmers concerned (rabbit, duck or pheasant farms —

chicken farms with diseases such as haemorrhagic enteritis…). The field (veterinarians and diagnostic laboratories) should gather the supporting data. The more obvious the disease impact on the target species and customers, the fewer the cases needed to evaluate the seriousness of the situation. For example: rabbit haemorrhagic disease (high percentages of mortality) versus variant infectious bronchitis (conditions causing only very slight mortality problems but having significant economic impact – feed conversion ratio…). It is very important that authorities have a flexible understanding of *"serious disease epidemic"*. Otherwise, this article cannot apply for "MUMS".

– Provisional use: unless the disease is eradicated or gone within a short period of time, the manufacturer proposing the answer to the problem should have a plan so that the vaccine is registered in a timely manner.

Authorisations for temporary use should be (in fact they are) reviewed regularly on the basis of epidemiology, pharmaco-vigilance and the progress of the manufacturer in its registration plan. It is quite right that authorities may cancel ATU if the answers from the manufacturer and the field on these points is not clear.

Technical data to be made available for the permission: (there are no details in E.U. Directive 81/852). We believe that the "data package" should not be fixed. It should depend on the urgency of the situation and the nature of the vaccine (strain, inactivated vaccine or not) based on an assessment of the risk versus the benefit of the use of the product. Authorities and manufacturers know the minimum criteria under which it is not possible to give permission. These criteria are detailed in Parts II and IV, and regard the safety of the strain (for example: extraneous agents, inactivation if the vaccine is inactivated, and reversion to virulence if it is a live vaccine…).

Although the E.U. guidelines must eventually be implemented as a registration plan is the logical step after any temporary authorisation, many issues can be temporarily addressed with the help of risk assessment tools. Already, many authorities are proceeding this way but there is no harmonised guidance for the risk/benefit assessment. We therefore suggest that such a guide is established by the authorities and the vaccine manufacturers.

Article 10 of E.U. Directive 2001/82EC states:

Where there is no authorized medicinal product for a condition, Member States may exceptionally, in particular to avoid causing ***unacceptable suffering*** *to the animals concerned, permit administration by a veterinarian or* ***under his/her direct personal responsibility to an animal or to a small number of animals on a particular holding****:*

a) *of a veterinary medicinal product authorised in the Member State concerned under this Directive or under Regulation (EEC) No 2309/93 for use in another animal species, or for another condition in the same species; or*

b) and c) articles do not concern vaccines

For the purposes of this paragraph, the phrase *"an animal or a small number of animals on a particular holding"* also covers pets, and shall be interpreted more flexibly for **minor or exotic animal species** which do not produce food.

This article can clearly be related to "MUMS". It introduces the notion of suffering and it is related to the personal responsibility of the veterinarian and limits the number of animals concerned. It allows the controlled use of "off-label" claims and to a great extent complements article 7 that mentions the case for vaccine registered in another State.

Article 26-third paragraph of E.U. Directive 2001/82EC states:

3. In exceptional circumstances, and following consultation with the applicant, an authorization may be granted subject to certain specific obligations, and subject to annual review, including:

- *The carrying out of further studies following the granting of authorization,*
- *The notification of adverse reactions to the veterinary medicinal product,*
- *These exceptional decisions may only be adopted for objective and verifiable reasons.*

This article is meant to give flexibility in the course of the registration process, allowing "MUMS" to be on the market when issues still to be resolved are not key aspects to a proper use of the vaccine. A timetable can be agreed with authorities and it allows the manufacturer to start selling the vaccine before the full registration work is carried out and paid for.

Conclusions

Flexibility is built in the "founding" directive for the registration of vaccines in the E.U. Authorities could use it more widely and without breaching the spirit of the E.U. registration system, provided a sound rationale is given and a risk/benefit assessment tool is widely used. We believe that the authorities, which are the most in favour of the flexible registration of "MUMS", should establish with the concerned manufacturers a guide for the steps to follow. This guide could serve as a model during the time when new technical and administrative requirements are set for "MUMS" at the E.U. level.

It is clear that this short-term flexibility, even if used well, will not suffice in the long term. Indeed, with the exception of some provisions, the law always requires that the totality of the work to be carried out eventually. In some circumstances, as explained earlier, this is not feasible from an economical point of view. We believe that more than the technical guidelines, the mutual recognition procedures are impractical for "MUMS". Except for article 7, all the flexibility given by the law is seen on a national level. As soon as we enter the MRP, the full "data package" is required and this constitutes a blocking point for applicants.

In all cases, any flexible system adapted to the situation of vaccines for minor use and minor species is based on trust between the authorities themselves and between the authorities and manufacturers.

Dr. J. de Foucauld, CEVA-Phylaxia, Szallàs u. 5, H-1107 Budapest, Hungary.
E-mail: jean. de-foucauld@ceva.com

Jungbäck C (ed): Consideration of Alternative Licensing Procedures for Vaccines for Minor Species, Minor Indications and Autogenous/Autologous Products.
Dev Biol. Basel, Karger, 2004, vol 117, pp 123-128.

Vaccine Use and Abuse: a Practitioner's Viewpoint

G.A. Moore

CPAC/American Veterinary Medicinal Association, Pembroke, VA, USA

Introduction

The worldwide production and sale of vaccines used in livestock and companion animal species is understandably closely regulated by government agencies. There must be some assurance that such products are safe and effective for the animals treated, and that there are no significant risks for persons administering such vaccines or consuming products derived from treated animals. However, from the standpoint of veterinarians and producers working with animal species generally considered to be of less commercial significance (minor species) or trying to control diseases with limited geographical distribution or simply low rates of occurrence (minor uses), the existing system does appear to limit vaccine availability. This paper attempts to summarize the current issues of vaccine availability in the United States; describes measures and actions taken to circumvent existing problems; and considers alternatives to improve the present situation with regard to vaccine availability especially for such minor species and minor uses.

Current Situation

In the United States, as in the rest of the world, many disparate groups have an interest in the availability and use of vaccines for the treatment and control of diseases in animals. Above all, these groups should have human safety as their overriding concern. The majority of them would also consider improvements in animal health, safety and production as a principal objective. Significant parties involved include: government regulatory agencies, primarily the Center for Veterinary Biologicals (CVB) of the United States Department of Agriculture

(USDA); biologicals manufacturers and their trade associations; animal owners and their representative producer/owner groups; veterinarians and their relevant professional associations; public interest groups; and legislators and lobbyists.

Despite their common aims, related to human safety and improved animal production issues, these groups can also have particular concerns that result in diametrically opposing objectives with respect to vaccine availability. Regulatory agencies might be unwilling to allow expanded use of a particular vaccine if such use would compromise a disease eradication programme in another species. Manufacturers might question the extent, and cost, of the testing required to modify the label of an existing vaccine to allow its use in an additional species. Given this myriad list of concerned groups, the existing system of regulation and production does function in a surprisingly effective manner and results in the licensing and marketing of many vaccines.

The availability of a vaccine for the control of a particular disease in any animal species is a function of the ability to develop, license, and manufacture a safe and effective product in a profitable manner. If one considers the so-called major species in the United States; designated by the Code of Federal Regulations (CFR) as cattle, horses, swine, chickens, turkeys, dogs, and cats, the availability of vaccines is quite satisfactory. Periodic complaints are made that the current approval process and regulations are too restrictive and costly and limit the development and marketing of products. However, vaccines, labelled for use in these species, against most of the economically significant diseases, are marketed. The existing system also appears to allow for the introduction of vaccines directed against entirely new diseases and the modification and reformulation of existing products in a timely fashion.

However, other vaccines, particularly those of benefit for minor uses or minor species, may be unavailable for a variety of reasons. For example, despite continuing research by universities, government agencies, and biologicals manufacturers, the development of an effective vaccine against a particular disease can be unsuccessful. A good example of this circumstance, at this time, is the retroviral infections of small ruminants, Ovine Progressive Pneumonia (OPP) and Caprine Arthritis and Encephalitis (CAE).

For some diseases an effective vaccine may exist, and even be licensed and manufactured, but because of the nature of the disease in the United States, government regulators restrict its use. Vaccines for *Bacillus anthracis* (anthrax), *Mycobacterium paratuberculosis* (Johne's disease), and *Brucella abortus* (Bang's disease) are all licensed and manufactured but their availability is limited. The use of the *Mycobacterium paratuberculosis* vaccine is restricted to cattle only in certain States and requires specific USDA approval before use due to prevailing regulatory efforts to control and potentially eradicate this disease. Similarly, the brucellosis vaccine is restricted to use in cattle and may only be administered by a federally accredited veterinarian.

Even if a safe and effective vaccine can be developed and licensed, the profitability of any such product is a, if not the, deciding factor in whether such an appropriately labelled product is made available on the market. If a biologicals manufacturer cannot justify the costs of developing, licensing, and marketing a vaccine designed to control a particular disease in a particular species, such a product is unlikely to be available. Profitability can even be a factor in the availability of an existing, appropriately licensed biological product. Because vaccines produced specifically for minor uses or minor species are by their nature in low demand, and so low profit, items, manufacturers will periodically displace production of such vaccines in favour of other, more profitable products. As a result such minor use or minor species vaccines may only be available at irregular intervals and unpredictable times. Such disruptions in supply can decrease the overall usefulness of a vaccine and potentially jeopardizes its long-term production and availability.

From the point of view of veterinarians and producers responsible for the health maintenance and overall management of animals designated as minor species, the existing system for vaccine licensing and production is imperfect because of the lack of approved vaccines for many economically significant diseases in these animals. In many cases the failure in this system is only emphasized by the availability of an appropriate, potentially effective vaccine which only lacks the incorporation of such species on to its label.

A partial list of such potentially useful vaccines for the control of significant diseases in minor species, particularly sheep and goats, in the United States at present would include:

The sheep vaccine for the control of caseous lymphadenitis (*Corynebacterium pseudotuberculosis* infection) is not labelled for goats despite the significant incidence of the disease in that species.

The sheep and goat vaccine for the control of bluetongue (orbivirus infection) might be useful in the management of farmed deer populations.

Several cattle and swine vaccines, used to control respiratory diseases resulting from a variety of viral and bacterial infections in these major species, could be beneficial in controlling disease outbreaks caused by identical or related organisms in certain minor species. Examples include mycoplasma pneumonias of sheep and goats; *Pasteurella spp.* infections in sheep, goats, and farmed deer species; and Parainfluenza-3 virus, upper airway infections in sheep.

Similarly, cattle and swine vaccines used to control gastro-intestinal infections, particularly *Escherichia coli*, associated with neonatal diarrhoea and death could be helpful in controlling the similar problems in sheep and goats.

Sheep vaccines, designed to control abortions caused by *Chlamydia psittaci* (Enzootic Abortion of Ewes) and *Campylobacter spp.* (Vibriosis), appear to be effective in controlling similar problems in goats. Cattle vaccines to control abortions caused by *Leptospira spp.*, similarly, should be effective in protecting both sheep and goats from comparable infections. While not a significant cause of abortions in sheep and goats, *Brucella abortus*, can be a problem in farmed deer species but, as discussed above, the USDA restricts the use of the available vaccine to cattle only.

Mycobacterium paratuberculosis infections or Johne's disease can also be a significant problem in herds and flocks of sheep, goats, llamas, alpacas, and farmed deer. The available vaccine would appear to be effective in controlling clinical expression of the disease in cattle with its associated loss in production and profitability. The vaccine's safety and efficacy in other ruminant species is largely untested in the United States and due to USDA-imposed restrictions its use in any species other than cattle is unlikely. While frustrating to owners and veterinarians attempting to control this disease in an affected flock, such restrictions, designed to limit seroconversion of uninfected animals, are justified given the USDA's current efforts to control the disease nationwide.

Lastly, several effective rabies vaccinations are available in the United States. While some are labelled for use in sheep, none is labelled for use in goats. Given the safety and efficacy of available vaccines in species included on their label (cats, dogs, sheep, cattle, horses, and ferrets) the expectation would be that they should be effective in protecting other species, particularly goats and camelids (specifically llamas and alpacas). Due to public health concerns and regulations concerning the disposition of unvaccinated animals following confirmed exposure to rabies, this lack of inclusion on the approved label is of particular concern to owners of such animals and their veterinarians.

Current Practices

To provide effective vaccination programmes to maintain healthy, productive, and profitable populations of animals, in the face of the described inadequacies in vaccine availability, owners, producers, and their veterinarians have had to resort to several optional measures. The first among these is the «off-label» or extralabel use of available biological products. As described above there are a number of vaccines available in the United States that are safe and effective in controlling diseases caused by similar, if not identical, infectious agents in other, major, species.

While little or no manufacturer-sponsored research to demonstrate the safety and efficacy of such use is available, it is still a widespread practice. In some situations producer groups or university researchers will conduct limited trials to evaluate the use of a particular vaccine in a particular group or species of animals. Over time, information on the apparent safety and efficacy, and occasionally the hazards, of such use is established. Such information is dispersed through producer group and practitioner association meetings or newsletters, and increasingly through Internet and Web postings and so becomes common knowledge. While such practices are a useful, if potentially dangerous, method of determining the safety of a particular product, an accurate determination of its efficacy really requires controlled studies which should at least involve titre and duration of immunity determinations, and clinical challenge trials.

Several concerns exist regarding such extralabel use of vaccines. Despite apparent widespread use, safety and especially efficacy issues are a potential problem. The question must always be asked as to how reliable is the source of the information. This has become an even greater worry with the rapid and widespread, Web-based, distribution of often misleading if not totally erroneous information. Although not required by current regulations, as it is for the extralabel use of pharmaceutical agents in animals, the extralabel use of biological products should ideally only be carried out under the auspices of a veterinary-client-patient-relationship.

From the veterinary practitioner standpoint, an added and significant concern is the issue of liability. The possibility of being held financially responsible for an unexpected or undesirable outcome following administration of a vaccine to an animal or group of animals is always a concern. If the species of animal so treated is not included in the label indications of that product the likelihood of successfully defending oneself against a liability claim would be considerably reduced. Even in situations where the owner is adequately advised as to the potential risks before such vaccine use, where the veterinarian involved is only a source of information regarding such use, or the veterinarian involved is only the supplier of the vaccine, a successful liability claim could be brought.

An alternative to gain access to appropriate vaccines is the use of foreign products. Given the economic significance and total population of some livestock species in other parts of the world, different countries may have effective, licensed vaccine products long before such a product is, if ever, marketed in the United States. For example, although equivalent products are now available here, for quite some time vaccines for caseous lymphadenitis and footrot in sheep (and goats) were widely available only in Commonwealth countries. Sheep and goat producers in the United States had ways of acquiring such products although the USDA discouraged the practice. Such use was based on information determined in a manner similar to that involved in extralabel use. But since the product being used had gone through an approval process in another country there was the added advantage of greater assurance of safety and efficacy. The regulatory agencies' concerns were based on discrepancies in standards of testing between the United States and the foreign countries involved.

A third alternative used to control diseases in the absence of effective, licensed vaccine is the use of autogenous vaccination. The USDA has provisions in their regulations that allow the production of autogenous vaccines under well-established guidelines. Complaints about these regulations, particularly those related to details of manufacturing, and isolation and identification of an organism used to produce a vaccine, are discussed with the USDA periodically. Biologicals manufacturers who specialize in the production of autogenous vaccines and large corporate livestock producers generally raise such complaints. In fact it can be relatively easy for an individual owner or producer, with or without veterinary involvement, to produce a vaccine for use in his or her own animals. The implied advantages to the use of autogenous vaccines include the more rapid development of a vaccine targeting a specific strain or newly emerging disease and in some circumstances a cost saving over the use of commercially available vaccines. While the USDA regulates the manufacture of autogenous vaccines, the proliferation of such production does raise a concern as to how that agency, with only finite resources, will continue to provide adequate supervision. Moreover, as the technology available for the modification of biological agents for the production of vaccines improves, will more detailed regulation be required to assure the overall safety of autogenous vaccine production and use.

Possible Improvements

It is unrealistic to imagine that veterinarians and owners involved with minor species production will ever be able to control all their disease problems through vaccination. First, not all diseases are amenable to control through vaccination. Second, the limited profit potential for biological products directed specifically at minor species will continue to make it unlikely that commercial manufacturers will devote much effort to the development and marketing of such vaccines. Third, the regulatory agencies have only finite resources to direct towards facilitating the development of new or the modification of existing products and labels to expand vaccine availability for use in minor species.

There are some alternatives to vaccination for disease control that could be considered. These would include reducing exposure to and risk of infection through environmental modification. Principally this would involve less intensive farming methods to improve environmental quality, decrease stress levels, and reduce the transmission of infectious agents. All such measures would however be likely to increase the cost of livestock production. Another alternative would be the use of additional medications to control disease transmission and severity. A third alternative would be genetic selection or possibly modification to improve animal health and productivity. While possibly being an effective way of controlling disease, it is unlikely that the public would universally accept any of these options. Vaccination as a method of disease control would in all likelihood be preferred.

To improve the existing situation with regard to vaccine availability for minor species, and to a lesser extent for minor uses, the following issues need to be examined. The «off-label» or extralabel use of vaccines requires that issues of human and animal safety be addressed. Some human safety issues could be considered by extrapolation from existing information in licensed species. If necessary, as with extralabel drug use, extended withdrawal times following vaccination could be instituted. An additional approach would be the use of extralabel vaccination in only certain livestock categories that are not likely to enter the human food chain imminently, if at all.

Similarly some animal safety issues could be considered by extrapolation from existing information in licensed species. Documentation of adverse reactions to extralabel vaccine use would also address animal safety issues, but would require that agencies and sites currently recording adverse events, report events in species other than those for which a product is licensed.

A significant source of information on extralabel use of vaccines could be data-generated for the licensing of products in foreign countries and records of product use after a licence is granted. Standards for licensing may not be identical to those in the United States but with continuing efforts directed at international harmonization, common standards could be considered. With the additional information provided by this documentation of extralabel use, relevant indications could be added to a vaccine label, to allow some form of provisional licensing of at least some major species products for use in minor species (or for minor uses). The addition of minor species information to labels would provide some assurance to the owners, producers, veterinarians, and the public that such use is safe and effective for all concerned.

Acknowledgements

Websites:

- Center for Veterinary Medicine, Food and Drug Administration
  http://www.fda.gov/cvm/default.html
- Center for Veterinary Biologicals
  http://www.aphisweb.aphis.usda.gov/vs/cvb/index.htm
- Sheepman Supply Company
  http://www.sheepman.com
- Colorado Serum Company
  http://www.colorado-serum, com/
- Fort Dodge Aanimal Health
  http://www.wyeth.com/divisions/fort_dodge. asp

Dr. G.A. Moore, CPAC/American Veterinary Medicinal Association, 159 Liberty Lane, Pembroke, VA 24136-3078, USA.
E-mail: torbeag@swva.net

Jungbäck C (eds): Consideration of Alternative Licensing Procedures for Vaccines for Minor Species, Minor Indications and Autogenous/Autologous Products.
Dev Biol. Basel, Karger, 2004, vol 117, p 129.

SESSION II (Part 2)

Vaccines for Minor Use and Minor Species

Necessary Changes in Legal Provisions

Moderator: *P. Jones* (EMEA)

Jungbäck C (ed): Consideration of Alternative Licensing Procedures for Vaccines for Minor Species, Minor Indications and Autogenous/Autologous Products.
Dev Biol. Basel, Karger, 2004, vol 117, pp 131-135.

Minor Species/Minor Indications: Legal Provisions, Definition Criteria and Policies to Be Considered

O. Papadopoulos

Department of Microbiology and Infectious Diseases, Faculty of Veterinary Medicine, Aristotle University, Thessaloniki, Greece

Abstract: The problem of availability of immunological products in minor species and minor indications/uses is complex and should be well defined. Data for species are available, but not for minor uses. "Case-by-case" decisions should be avoided, as far as possible. The following categories can be recognized: (a) a vaccine has not been authorized anywhere; (b) a vaccine is authorized for major species/indications only; (c) an authorized vaccine exists in another Member State and (d) a vaccine has been withdrawn. Old, well established products, with limited data for an updated dossier could be the problem in categories "c" and "d". Proposed measures and incentives include: "cascade" (not recommended), human orphan-like drug policy, provisional authorization, acceptance of bibliographical data (if justified), procedural and financial assistance. Standards of quality, safety and efficacy cannot be minimized, but specific tests can be considered.

INTRODUCTION

The problem of availability of veterinary medicines for minor species and minor indications is well recognized in Europe by the veterinary profession, but also by the regulative and legislative authorities (Communication of the Commission to Council and Parliament 5/12/2000: Availability of veterinary medicinal products COM (2000) 806.final). The main cause is known: the small market with the consequent lack of commercial interest. There is no direct solution, but only indirect measures.

Problem Identification

Practising veterinarians, when asked for examples of MUMS vaccines, identify vaccines that have not been authorized anywhere, or are authorized for major species/uses only, or in another Member State, or vaccines that have been withdrawn.

Current Situation

Background

The European legislation on MUMS originated from the above- mentioned « Communication of the Commission » in 2000. The current policy is outlined in the draft document « Position paper regarding availability for products for minor uses and minor species (MUMS) », produced by the Committee for Veterinary Medicinal Products (CVMP), due to be finalized after consultation by interested parties in 2004 (EMEA/CVMP/477/03-Consultation). It is not the purpose of this presentation to analyse this position paper. However, it will be taken as a reference, as it is intended to shape European policies for the years to come. Priority has been given to pharmaceuticals, with extrapolation of existing MRLs from major species. Licensing applications are expected to follow. For immunological products, the policy is still under development.

Definition of minor species

Based on the experience gained during the extrapolation of MRLs, animal population number thresholds were taken as a basis for defining minor species. Global animal numbers across Europe were considered, instead of numbers within Member States (15 million for mammalian species, with the exception of rabbits and dairy sheep, 200 million for poultry and 100,000 tons for fish produced). Based on these threshold values, the following species were defined as major:

- Cattle (dairy and meat animals)
- Sheep (meat-animals) (?)
- Pigs
- Chickens (including laying hens)
- *Salmonidae*
- Dogs
- Cats

As a consequence all other species are classed as minor. This classification can apply to immunologicals, with the exception of sheep. Differentiation between milk-producing and meat-only sheep is necessary for setting MRLs, but is irrelevant to vaccines. In addition, confusion can be caused if flocks of milk or meat-producing breeds are in the same area.

Definition of minor indication/use

In the human sector the definition of minor use is based on the number of cases treated. This type of epidemiological data for animal diseases is not reliably collected. Similarly, the option to establish a threshold based on product sale values is not feasible, because these products are not marketed. Case-by-case solutions are not desirable, but are unavoidable. The only practical approach, at present, seems to identify a minor use once the company has submitted documentation to support a minor use of a product. The importance of the product in question, to avoid animal suffering, production losses due to non-availability of treatment, as well as estimates of future market sales, should be taken into account. The minor use approvals should only be considered by one single expert body (see : human orphan drug policy). Once experience has been gained, criteria could be defined. Another approach could be that candidate uses (e.g. anthrax in pigs) are proposed by National Authorities and designated by the single expert body.

Orphan drug policy for human use

This policy is intended for rare diseases, defined as « a life-threatening or chronically debilitating condition affecting not more than five in 10,000 persons ». A Committee on Orphan Medicinal Products (COMP) has been established to examine applications. It is based on a two-step procedure : designation, based on data submitted by the company, and authorization. Incentives including fee waivers, scientific advice, market exclusivity, community research opportunities (Reg. 141/2000, Reg. 847/2000). Presently, 164 products have been designed as orphans (no vaccines) and 11 were authorized. Specific epidemiological data are missing for animal diseases but could be useful as a model.

Cascade principle (extra label use)

Extra label use of products authorized for other species, or for another condition, is permitted in exceptional cases and for a small number of animals in a particular holding, under the personal responsibility of a veterinarian (Dir. 2001/82/EC, article 10). This provision is applied extensively, but for vaccines, safety and efficacy risk concerns exist, due to different susceptibility and pathogens or serotypes. Examples are feline/canine parvovirus in the past, vaccinations of quails, ostriches and monkeys. Also, the use in goats of paratuberculosis and contagious agalactia vaccines authorized for sheep.

Provisional authorization

In specific situations a provisional authorization may be given, with the provision of post-authorization commitments (Reg. 2309/93). It is an important but little used provision, mainly because a full authorization must follow.

Line extension

In the form of « extrapolation » it has been already applied in the set-up of MRLs from major to minor species (Dir. 2001/82/EC). It could be applied in immunologicals for the extension from major to minor species. Normally, only safety and efficacy data are required.

Specific authorizations

Provisions for specific importation for field or experimental use.

Emergency vaccines

In emergency situations of epizootic diseases, unauthorized vaccines may be used by National Authorities, after informing the Commission (Dir. 2001/82/EC). It is not applicable to common conditions. There is little regulation regarding quality, safety and efficacy.

Autogenous vaccines

These are defined as « Inactivated immunological products which are manufactured from pathogens and antigens obtained from an animal or animals from a holding and used for treatment of that animal or the animals of that holding in the same locality » (Dir. 2001/82/EC). This subject was extensively discussed in the first part of the present meeting. Autogenous vaccines are extremely important for the MUMS problem and their use is increasing. Their production and use is regulated by Member States. As the free movement of animals and between Member States is increasing and animal management conditions are changing, problems arise. Questions that should be answered are : for antigens, should they be bacterial, viral, inactivated, live ? For production : GMP, site licence, product licence, no licence at all ? New definitions are needed for holding, locality, multi-site units, and epidemiological unit.

Policies to Be Considered

General incentives

Quality : Reduced requirements not acceptable.

Safety : Limited possibility for reduced requirements, e.g. target species double dose or environmental impact in line extensions.

Efficacy : Reduced requirements possible, if justified (discussed by the speakers following). Provisional authorization with commitments.

Bibliographical documentation : May be accepted, if justified. Applicable especially for old, well-established products.

Financial incentives : Fee waivers, free advice, market exclusivity, specific research opportunities, have been already discussed by other speakers.

A vaccine has not been authorized anywhere

Description : Although information on certain experimental vaccines has been published, there are no applications for licensing. The cause : high costs and uncertainties for developing and licensing new vaccines, when low financial returns are envisaged.

Policies to be considered : General incentives, orphan-like policy, provisional authorizations, autogenous vaccines.

Vaccine is already authorized for major species only

Description: Applications for line extensions to MUMS are not submitted, because new safety and efficacy studies are required. In certain cases different pathogens or serotypes are involved.

Policies to be considered: General incentives, line extension.

Vaccine is already authorized in another a Member State

Description: Mutual recognition applications are not submitted. Sometimes, well-established products are involved, with limited data for an updated dossier.

Policies to be considered: General incentives, advice for an updated dossier, specific importation.

Vaccine was authorized but has been withdrawn

Description: May be old, well-established products, with limited data for an update dossier. Worst-case scenario.

Policies to be considered: General incentives for a new application. The established methodology may be used for the production of autogenous vaccine.

Conclusion

The availability problem for vaccines for minor species/indications can be addressed only by a variety of alternative complementary measures. The basic requirement is an acceptable level for quality, safety and efficacy.

References

- EMEA/CVMP Documents: http://www.emea.eu.int
- EC Regulations and Directives: http://www.eu.int (Links)

Dr. O. Papadopoulos, Faculty of Veterinary Medicine, Aristotle University, GR-54124 Thessaloniki, Greece.
E-mail: orestisp@vet.auth.gr

Jungbäck C (ed): Consideration of Alternative Licensing Procedures for Vaccines for Minor Species, Minor Indications and Autogenous/Autologous Products.
Dev Biol. Basel, Karger, 2004, vol 117, pp 137-140.

Vaccines for Minor Use and Minor Species: Technical Difficulties to Solve and Consequences in Legal Definitions

P. Vannier

AFSSA, Ploufragan, France

Abstract: To identify the difficulties of the problem and to try to find some solutions with their consequences in legal provisions, different aspects have to be considered: the possible definitions of minor species and minor indications and the limits of such definitions, the present applicable directives and possible modifications induced by extrapolation of technical results, by reduction of requirements.
According to the complexity of the problem, a pragmatic approach with a certain flexibility, founded on a case-by-case assessment, seems to be necessary.
The basis of the CVMP position paper regarding the availability of products for minor uses and minor species mainly focused on medicinal products and MRLs is interesting to consider in the case of vaccines, in the light of technical requirements of Title II of EU Directive 2001/82/EC.
Even if definitions of minor species and minor uses are needed to give a legal basis for the problem, they have limits and some examples will be given. Reduction of requirements and extrapolation seem possible in a relatively easy way when data are available for major use and major species. A reduction of requirements is much more difficult to set up when such data are not available. Requirements for quality, safety and efficiency will be assessed including the indications of notifiable diseases. When all these aspects have been considered, it is essential to avoid a disharmonised approach from the National Regulatory Authorities. So, the possibilities of a specific legal framework on « Minor Uses and Minor Species » and a centralised procedure for marketing authorisations have to be discussed.

Introduction

In the present situation, there is a clear lack of availability of vaccines for minor use and for minor species, creating a major problem in animal health. There are certainly two main reasons for the problem: the market is too restricted to be profitable considering the high level of requirements, which involve a high cost in research and development for new vaccines or extension of claims for existing vaccines.

State of the problem: possible solutions

It does not seem possible to act directly on the size of the market or to give the exclusivity of a market to one company for a certain period; finding the solution to establishing a consensus between competitors would be difficult.

It seems easier to act on the cost of research and development resulting from the level of requirements and the need for compliance of the marketing application (MA) file with the present regulation. Cost also results from the number and type of assays to be carried out to elaborate a MA. As a consequence, solutions can only be found if there is a certain decrease in the level of requirements and/or on a flexible approach, by working by analogy or extrapolation of data on a case-by- case basis and on risk analysis. Such an approach has to be complemented with feedback information from the field linked to an effective vaccino-vigilance and a conditional licence.

However, at the European level, there is a need to create the basis of a harmonised approach, founding the process on a legal basis with a clear definition of the framework and of minor uses and minor species.

Different Aspects of the Problem to Be Considered

Need for legal definitions

One interesting work may be used as a basis for the approach in finding a reasonable legal definition [1]. Even if the vaccines have nothing to do with MRLS (maximum residue limits), thoughts expressed in that document are interesting to consider. "Minor uses" is defined as a minor indication in a major species. "Minor species" is defined by the threshold of animal numbers in the EU.

In some cases, factors other than animal numbers have been used to define specified animal species as minor. These include, for instance, a low economic value of the single animal (e. g. the honey bee). But these definitions have limits; a minor species can be minor in one member state and major in another.

From the CVMP position paper, major food-producing species are: cattle, sheep (meat animals), pigs, chickens, including laying hens, and Salmonids. All other animal species are classified, by default, as minor: rabbits, bees, sheep (dairy) and goats. But turkeys are major in France and minor in other countries.

For minor uses, it seems to be more difficult to define criteria; this has to be done considering that, for example, certain diseases can have a low prevalence in a major species. So, it is difficult to establish a threshold.

Proposal of practical solutions

From the analysis of the difficulties, principles can be set up for founding the legal basis.

The most practical approach seems to be the risk analysis on a case-by-case basis. But it is necessary, as a pre-requisite, to manage the risk. There are two different situations: when a product exists in a major species and can be used in minor species, when there is no specific product available. So the working principles could be to proceed by analogies, using the results from one species to other ones under conditions in which the species can be considered as close as possible from the phylogenetical point of view.

It is also possible to work by extrapolation from the results from one species to the assessment of the effects of the vaccine in other species. For example, if data on serology/challenge are available in one species, serology could be sufficient to assess the efficacy, (not only activity) in other species.

Examples

What kind of risk analysis can be done on Newcastle disease vaccines in pigeons which is a major problem in a minor species? It is important to favour aqueous adjuvanted vaccines to prevent problems during flight, taking into account limited assays for safety and activity. But what kind of vaccinal strain can be used: homologous? heterologous? Decisions and acceptability will be based on the knowledge of certain parameters such as the cross protection induced. But, with a limited number of assays, the validation of the tests will depend on the pertinence of the protocol such as the choice of the challenge strain which has to express a high virulence whereas, in several assays, a lack of pathogenicity can be observed.

Assays to be performed for the MA

It seems necessary to elaborate a legal basis which allows long-term views to be supplied to the manufacturers. The basis is EU directive 2001/82, titre II: IVMPs.

Considering the analytical part, the same documents could be used from major species MAs to analogous minor species MAs. Concerning part F related to controls on finished products, the assays performed on major target species could be accepted for minor proximal species. Requirements have to be maintained at a relatively high level for quality.

Considering the safety part, it is necessary to try to explain the European approach; the assessment of the safety of vaccines is done through the cumulative results of different assays to try to establish as precisely as possible the biological properties of a vaccine.

So as a principle, in a MA, some assays performed on the target major species could be accepted for minor species by analogy. Assays could be limited to ones related to extreme conditions. If the results are acceptable, these assays could be sufficient to build up the file. For example, the inactivated vaccines could be tested with a double dose at the minimal age of claims and the other assays performed on major species could be accepted by extrapolation. For live vaccines, there is a need for a real risk analysis on a case-by-case basis. In consequence, assays such as reversion of virulence, dissemination would be carried out only on major species and not on minor ones. Risk analysis would be the support of the approach to limit the number of assays. When a totally new product needs to be developed in minor species, considering the efficacy part, the assessment of a product used on minor species could be founded on extrapolation and analogy.

The protection induced in minor species could be assessed by comparing the antibody titres obtained after vaccination of minor species with the ones observed in major species before challenge. The challenges would therefore be done in limited conditions. For example, poultry Newcastle Disease vaccines were tested in different species of game birds [2]. The safety of the vaccines was correct for pheasants and red-grey partridges. However, it appeared difficult to assess the efficacy of the vaccines on red partridges because of a lower sensitivity to the challenge strain.

In addition, the proposal is not to do any field studies or to base the assessment (safety, activity measured by serology) only on field studies. In the case of a new product, limited assays could be accepted, founded on activity rather than on efficacy.

In summary, the principles to solve the problem of vaccines for minor species would be to deliver a marketing authorization from data collected mainly on proximal major species with limited assays on target minor species.

In some cases, it could be very useful that additional assays could be performed by public laboratories which would be included in the assessment of the vaccine; in that situation a coordination would be necessary: from EMEA/EDQM? From EU DG research or enterprise?

Vaccino-vigilance

As a complement of these limited assays, it is fundamental to implement an efficient follow-up of sampling vaccinated minor species herds after marketing authorization. This implies the creation of a provisional or conditional licensing procedure including immediate suspension if a problem occurs.

Conclusion

From the previous analysis, it appears that several solutions exist to solve that problem. The main obstacle could be the acceptance at the EU level of a real management of the risk.

However, animal health is really faced with an emergency situation given a decrease in the availability of vaccines, a monopoly of a few manufacturers and a permanent decrease in the number of manufacturers, with a drastic change in the policy of investment which could create a dramatic problem in the future.

References

1 EMEA/CMVP/477/03. Position paper regarding availability of products from minor uses and minor species (MUMs).

2 Guittet M, Le Coq H, Picault JP, Morin Y: Maladie de Newcastle chez le gibier (faisans et perdrix): essai de prévention avec différents types de vaccin. Deuxièmes Journées de la Recherche Avicole, Tours, 8-10 Avril 1997. 1997, pp 107-110.

Dr. P. Vannier, AFSSA, B.P. 53, F-22440 Ploufragan, France.
E-mail: p.vannier@ploufragan.afssa.fr

Jungbäck C (ed): Consideration of Alternative Licensing Procedures for Vaccines for Minor Species, Minor Indications and Autogenous/Autologous Products.
Dev Biol. Basel, Karger, 2004, vol 117, pp 141-143.

Vaccines for Minor Use/Minor Species (MUMS) in the European Union

D. Mackay

Institute for Animal Health, Pirbright Laboratory, Woking, Surrey, U.K. (formerly of the Veterinary Medicines Directorate, Addlestone, Surrey)

The issue of the availability of veterinary vaccines has been much discussed since the introduction of harmonised Community pharmaceutical legislation led to a reduction in the range of products available. Initiatives have been launched at Community and national level to attempt to address the issue, to date with little success in terms of actually increasing the number or range of products on the market. This article attempts to define the issues that need to be faced in identifying solutions to the problem in relation specifically to immunological veterinary medicinal products (IVMPs) and goes on to identify legislative or policy changes that would need to be introduced to effect these solutions.

The current pharmaceutical directive, 2001/82/EC, has a number of specific provisions intended to increase the range of products available, specifically in the veterinary pharmaceutical armoury,

Art. 4 – permits Member States to exempt from the requirements of the Directive autogenous/autologous products i.e. those derived from antigens obtained from the premises on which the product is used. Such products, while useful, are small-scale, niche products that can never address the wider issues of availability.

Art. 7 – permits the use of products authorised in other Member States in accordance with the Directive and is intended for short-term use to allow access to medicines that are available elsewhere within the Community than the Member State concerned, 'where the health situation so requires'.

Art. 8 – permits the use of unauthorised IVMPs in the event of a serious disease epidemic. Again, this is intended as a short-term, emergency measure to allow access to unauthorised vaccines where the risks of importing and/or using such a product are outweighed by the potential consequences, in terms of animal disease, of not doing so. This provision has been used by Member States, and the Commission, to permit the use of unauthorised vaccines against foot-and-mouth disease, bluetongue and avian influenza. Although clearly intended to permit use under emergency circumstances, this provision is also used as the legal basis for procuring and storing stocks of unauthorised antigens and vaccines against OIE list A diseases in advance of need. This policy should be reviewed as it would seem reasonable that stocks laid down in advance of need should comply fully with pharmaceutical legislation and be assessed against the same criteria as any other vaccine.

Art. 10 – permits the use of the prescribing 'Cascade' to allow access to products authorised in other species, in man or prepared extemporaneously. This provision is widely used and allows access to essential medicines. However, from the veterinarian's perspective, it is bureaucratic to administer and is often not well understood by animal owners who are required to give informed consent. In addition, it could be considered to act as a disincentive to authorisation in minor species, as products already authorised in major species can legally be used in minor species, where appropriate, without the manufacturer having to go through the expense of authorisation.

Art. 26 – permits Licensing Authorities to issue conditional/provisional authorisations in exceptional circumstances and following consultation with the applicant. This permissive provision is not applied consistently between Member States and has never been used to permit provisional authorisation through the Centralised Procedure. In principle, the provision allows an authorisation to be granted in those situations where it is difficult, for a variety of reasons, to generate full efficacy data (or, more rarely, safety data) before authorisation. The requirement for annual review makes the procedure cumbersome for both manufacturers and Licensing Authorities to administer and a transparent, predictable and consistent procedure for authorisation of MUMS products would be preferable to extending use of this provision.

From the descriptions above it is clear that there are already legal provisions intended to address the availability issue for all species and uses, including MUMS. However, it is equally clear that the measures currently in place are inadequate as farmers and veterinarians in practice, who constitute the main user communities, are emphatic that more needs to be done to make a wider range of vaccines, and possibly other IVMPs, available.

There are very few measures included within the current review of pharmaceutical legislation that will have a major impact on availability and, indeed, some proposed amendments have the potential to have an adverse impact. The proposed amendments will 'open up' the prescribing cascade and will clarify the situation with regard to permitting the use of active ingredients not included in Annexes I, II or III of Directive 2377/90 in products authorised for horses not intended for human consumption. However, the proposed requirement for all products authorised for food-producing species to be prescription-only medicines could severely affect their availability without being of obvious benefit in terms of protecting consumers. There are no specific measures to define MUMS medicinal products or introduce a specific route to authorisation for these products, as exists for human orphan medicinal products.

Experience with the human orphan drugs policy in the U.S.A., and now within the EU, suggests that a two-pronged approach needs to be adopted. The first is to create incentives for manufacturers to develop MUMS products. This could be by providing extended periods of data protection, by providing scientific advice on regulatory issues free of charge, by reducing the fees charged for registration, and by assisting manufacturers to fill data gaps through the provision of funds through appropriate research and development funding. The second is to reduce the regulatory burden as far as possible by creating a transparent procedure for conditional/provisional licensing, by minimising data requirements as far as possible while retaining an adequate level of assurance of safety to the animal, to the user and to the environment, by accepting or sourcing data from sources other than the applicant and by permitting access to the Centralised Procedure for all MUMS products.

Making progress on the MUMS availability issue within the EU will require active participation from all stakeholders in the process. These stakeholders comprise (i) the EU Commission, in defining a clear MUMS policy and, where necessary, introducing the legislative and procedural changes that are necessary to implement it; (ii) manufacturers, in being prepared to investigate the market potential for MUMS products actively and to look at innovative ways in which regulatory requirements might be met and (iii) from the regulators, particularly the CVMP and its working parties, in looking critically at the data requirements for MUMS products and how these might reasonably be reduced without materially increasing risk. There is little prospect of reducing data requirements without a fundamental change in approach to risk management. Currently the entire regulatory process is based on risk reduction, and usually risk elimination, through the provision of data. If data requirements are to be significantly reduced, regulators, and the user community, must be prepared to tolerate a higher degree of risk in that data might be substituted by informed risk quantification, mitigation and, in some cases, risk acceptance.

Dr. D.K.J. Mackay, Institute for Animal Health, Pirbright Laboratory, Ash Road, Pirbright, Woking, Surrey GU24 0NF, United Kingdom.
E-mail: david.mackay@bbsrc.ac.uk

Jungbäck C (ed): Consideration of Alternative Licensing Procedures for Vaccines for Minor Species, Minor Indications and Autogenous/Autologous Products.
Dev Biol. Basel, Karger, 2004, vol 117, p 145.

SESSION II (Part 3)

Vaccines for Minor Use and Minor Species

Legal Basis, Definitions, Need for Availability and the Role of Conditional Licences: Authorities' Point of View

Moderator: *M. Moos* (PEI)

Jungbäck C (ed): Consideration of Alternative Licensing Procedures for Vaccines for Minor Species, Minor Indications and Autogenous/Autologous Products.
Dev Biol. Basel, Karger, 2004, vol 117, pp 147-152.

Regulation of Conditionally Licensed Biologicals in the United States

R.E. Hill

Center for Veterinary Biologics, USDA, Animal and Plant Health Inspection Service, Veterinary Services, Ames, IA, USA

Key words: Veterinary, vaccine, conditional licence, regulatory, minor use, emergency, licensing

Abstract: The Virus-Serum-Toxin Act of 1913 (21 US Code 151-159) provides the legal basis for the regulation of veterinary biologicals in the United States and the United States Department of Agriculture's Center for Veterinary Biologics (CVB) has the regulatory authority for the issuing of licences and permits for such products. The law was intended to establish standards and control the importation of products into the United States and the distribution of products interstate assuring the purity, safety, potency, and efficacy of veterinary biological products. Under certain specific circumstances, product licences may be issued in the United States under expedited procedures which assure purity, safety, and a "reasonable expectation" of efficacy. These conditional licences may be authorized to meet an emergency condition, limited market, local situation, or other special circumstances, and provide valuable tools for veterinarians and consumers in improving animal health.

INTRODUCTION

Federal regulation of veterinary biological products in the United States began in 1913 with the passage of the Virus-Serum-Toxin Act by the U.S. Congress. The United States Department of Agriculture's Center for Veterinary Biologics (CVB) is responsible for regulating veterinary biological products (including diagnostics). The law was intended to establish standards and control the importation of products into the United States and the distribution of products interstate assuring the purity, safety, potency, and efficacy of veterinary biological products. A combination of regulatory oversight before and after licensing assures the availability of pure, safe, potent, and effective veterinary biologicals to veterinarians and animal owners. Under certain specific circumstances, product licences may be issued under expedited procedures which assure purity, safety, and a "reasonable expectation" of efficacy. These conditional licences may be authorized to meet an emergency condition, limited market, local situation, or other special circumstance. The requirements for conditional licences are unique, yet are based on the same regulatory framework as conventionally licensed biological products except for completion of host animal testing or potency test development. The regulatory framework for licensing and basic criteria to qualify an individual product for licensing is described below to provide the basis for the discussion on specialized requirements for conditional licences.

Regulatory Framework

The Virus-Serum-Toxin Act of 1913 (21 US Code 151-159) provides the legal basis for the regulation of veterinary biologicals in the United States. The law was amended in 1985 by the Food Security Act to include the distribution of all veterinary biologicals (both interstate and intrastate) in the United States, as well as those intended for export. Administrative regulations and standards appear in Title 9, Code of Federal Regulations (9 CFR) Parts 101-118 with additional programme guidance found in Center for Veterinary Biologics Notices, Veterinary Services Memoranda, General Licensing Considerations and other guidance documents. Veterinary biological products are defined in the regulations as "all viruses, serums, toxins (excluding substances that are selectively toxic to micro-organisms; e.g., antibiotics), or analogous products at any stage of production, shipment, distribution, or sale, which are intended for use in the treatment of animals and which act primarily through the direct stimulation, supplementation, enhancement, or modulation of the immune system or immune response". This includes, but is not limited to, vaccines, bacterins, allergens, antibodies, antitoxins, toxoids, immunostimulants, certain cytokines, antigenic or immunizing components of live organisms, and diagnostic components which are of natural or synthetic origin, or which are derived from synthesizing or altering various substances or components of substances such as micro-organisms, genes or genetic sequences, carbohydrates, proteins, antigens, allergens, or antibodies.

Conventional Product Licensing Requirements

Pre-licensing data evaluation procedures are designed to assess the purity, safety, potency, and effectiveness of each product and support all product label claims. In order to fulfil these criteria, data from all phases of product development are evaluated against these key elements. This spectrum of evaluation includes complete characterization and identification of seed material and ingredients, laboratory and host animal safety and efficacy studies, demonstration of stability, and monitoring of field performance. Specific purity, safety, potency, and efficacy requirements are as follows:

Purity

All product components and ingredients must meet standards of purity and quality. Master Seed, Master Cell Stock, Primary Cells, ingredients of animal origin, and final products must be tested and shown to be free of extraneous micro-organisms. Eggs used in the production of biological products must be acquired from specific-pathogen-free flocks. The purity and identification of Master Seed and Master Cell are confirmed by testing at the CVB. In addition to the first serials (batches of completed product) prepared under licence, a random sample of serials are subjected to pre-release purity testing at the CVB to verify manufacturer's quality assurance/quality control on the final product.

Safety

Products must be shown to be safe through a combination of safety evaluations. Master Seeds and Master Cell Stocks must be fully identified and characterized. Production passage levels (limits) are established for both seeds and cells. Master Seeds for live products are tested for shed, spread, and reversion to virulence through back passage studies in the host animal. Following a minimum of five passages in the host, recovered isolates are fully characterized using the same procedures used for the Master Seed. Demonstration of an acceptable level of attenuation must be shown. Other safety studies are required as appropriate (e.g., use in pregnant animals, environmental safety, or adjuvants in products for food-producing animals which must be approved in consultation with the USDA Food Safety and Inspection Service). Field safety studies designed to detect unexpected reactions that may not have been detected in product development are required before licensing. Host animal tests are conducted at a variety of geographical sites using large numbers of susceptible animals representing all ages and husbandry practices for which the product is intended. Final products are subjected to safety testing primarily through in vivo animal tests.

Efficacy

All products must be shown to be effective according to the claims indicated on the label. Efficacy and product immunogenicity are generally demonstrated by statistically valid host animal vaccination-challenge studies. The following general considerations are applied to efficacy studies:

- Immunogenicity studies must be conducted using minimum levels of antigen at the highest passage level from the Master Seed that is permitted for production.
- The product must be prepared in production facilities on a scale representative of normal production.
- Challenge methods and criteria for evaluating protection will vary with the immunizing agent but in general, tests are conducted under controlled conditions using sero-negative animals of the youngest age recommended on the label.
- The duration of immunity data is required for some existing products (e.g., rabies) and for all newly licensed antigens.
- Field efficacy studies may be considered where laboratory animal challenge models are not well established. Similarly, serological data may be used to establish efficacy only when serology is indicative of protection.
- Data are required for each species for which the product is recommended and for each route, dose, and regimen of administration.

- For products with two or more fractions (components), data demonstrating no antigenic interference are required.
- Stability studies are required to set the expiry date on the label.
- Potency tests correlated to host animal vaccination and designed to measure the relative strength of each serial must be developed before licensing. In addition, each serial shall be formulated and tested before marketing to ensure effectiveness and reproducibility of activity (potency) according to standards set at the time of licensing. Generally, this is accomplished through established laboratory animal or in vitro minimum potency levels using microbiological counts or virus titrations.

Licensing data should be developed and submitted for licensing in a logical sequence representing successive steps in product development (e.g., Master Seed purity and identity, laboratory safety, immunogenicity, initial production serials [usually three], purity, safety, potency testing, and field safety). All data generated in product development are required to be reported to the CVB. Following receipt and evaluation of the data described above, products are eligible for licensing. Additional steps (not described herein) include approval of labelling, confirmatory testing, pre-licence inspection, and production method approval.

Conditional Product Licence Requirements

Conditional licences are authorized under very specialized circumstances to meet an emergency condition, limited market, local situation, or other special circumstance. This process allows the licensing of products to:

1) respond quickly to make products available during emerging disease situations;
2) license products for minor species or other limited markets that may not otherwise be available due to the cost of product development; and
3) license products where host animal efficacy studies have not been completed to the standard for conventionally licensed products, or where potency studies have not been established for serial testing.

Licences are issued under an expedited procedure which assures purity and safety, and a reasonable expectation of efficacy of the products involved. With conditionally licensed products, all the relevant requirements for purity, safety and identity must be met. Efficacy studies must be conducted to the extent that they provide confidence that the product is reasonably efficacious.

Conditional Product Licence Restrictions

Preparation of products under a conditional licence must be in compliance with all applicable regulations and standards. In addition, they also contain certain restrictions as a specification of licensing. Administrative regulations and standards appear in the 9 CFR, Part 102.6.

Licence expiry

The preparation of the conditionally licensed biological may be limited to a predetermined time period which is established at the time of licensing. A one-year expiry date is usually established. Before re-issuing, the manufacturer must demonstrate acceptable progress towards completion of host animal testing or potency test development. Product licences may be re-issued when substantiated data support progress towards a conventional licence.

Restricted distribution or use

Additional conditions on the licence restrict distribution to the extent necessary to ensure that the product will meet the basic criteria for issuing the conditional licence. Common restrictions include:

- For use by a veterinarian only.
- For use by or under the supervision of a veterinarian.
- Distribution in each State shall be limited to authorized recipients designated by proper State officials, under such additional conditions as these authorities may require.
- Re-issuing of this licence shall be considered in accordance with 9CFR Part 102.6.
- The licensee shall demonstrate acceptable progress toward completion of host animal efficacy and potency test studies in accordance with acceptable protocols filed with the Center for Veterinary Biologics before re-issuing.
- The following statement shall appear on all labels: This product licence is conditional. Efficacy and potency test studies in progress.
- Trade names shall not be used with this product.
- Marketing and promotional materials «restricted». (See comments for specific restriction.)
- This licence will terminate < specify date or duration > year from the date of issuing.
- Unusual conditions or adverse events linked to vaccinated animals are to be reported to the Center for Veterinary Biologics within five working days.
- Domestic distribution and use shall be under the supervision or control of USDA, APHIS, Veterinary Services, as part of an official USDA animal disease control programme.
- For use in «specified species» only. (See comments for species.)

Licence name and labelling

Only the Federally designated true name may be used in association with the product. A trade name may not be used on the label or in the advertising. Product labels are required to contain information on the conditional status of the licence.

Uniqueness

Conditional licences may only be issued for products that are truly unique (i.e., those that are not under conventional licences).

Summary

Vaccination is recognized worldwide as a valuable tool in controlling animal disease and vaccines have played an important role in a wide spectrum of disease eradication and control efforts. Because of these successes, vaccines are commonly considered during times of emerging or emergency animal disease situations, or for use in alternate species (off-label use). The range of products that is available for such uses is not always available due to limited markets, qualification difficulties, or costs of development.

Availability of products for minor species or limited markets will continue to be a concern, outbreaks will continue to occur wherever animals exist, diseases will continue to emerge worldwide, and users and animal health authorities will continue to be faced with challenges related to the use of vaccine under these conditions. In the United States, conditionally licensed products provide a means of making quality biologicals available for these scenarios. While the foundation for development and use of products in minor species, limited markets, or emerging and emergency situations remains focused on product purity, safety, potency, and efficacy, regulatory authorities and regulations authorizing the marketing of veterinary biologicals must be flexible enough to allow products to become available for such purposes. In addition, there must be incentives for research and development by biologicals manufacturers in order to have products available for emerging animal health situations, local situations, or limited markets. Conditional licences, and the marketing of products that are pure, safe, and expected to be effective, provide an incentive for research and development and a mechanism for the availability of such products.

Dr. R.E. Hill, Jr., Center for Veterinary Biologics, USDA, Animal and Plant Health Inspection Service, Veterinary Services, Suite 104, 510 South 17th Street, Ames, IA 50010, USA.
E-mail: rick.e.hill@aphis.usda.gov

Jungbäck C (ed): Consideration of Alternative Licensing Procedures for Vaccines for Minor Species, Minor Indications and Autogenous/Autologous Products.
Dev Biol. Basel, Karger, 2004, vol 117, pp 153-158.

Consideration of Alternative Licensing Procedures for Vaccines for Minor Species, Minor Indications and Autogenous/Autologous Products

P.G.H. Jones

Veterinary Medicines & Inspections, EMEA, London, U.K.

Legal Basis for Authorisation of Medicines in the EU

It is often reported that the regulatory process is seen to be too vigorous, too demanding and often too lengthy, so that it provides little incentive to develop products for minor uses and minor species that are the topic of this conference. In addition to the regulatory processes themselves as enshrined in EU legislation, we have to take account of political pressure and society values, as well as the pressures from the animal health industry, to provide products for the veterinarians, who are charged with a duty of care for the minor species that are the subject of discussion. However, it is imperative that whatever solutions may be found to make the provision of products and vaccines in particular for minor species easier, there is always a requirement to safeguard consumer health and safety; having to take regard of a system that for many years has worked extremely well bringing safe products into the market-place.

There are two main routes for authorisation of veterinary medicinal products in the EU. The first is the centralised route governed by Council Regulation 2309/93, which came into force on 1 January 1995 with the establishment of the European Medicines Evaluation Agency in London. This procedure is compulsory for all products, which meet the criteria set out in Part A of the Annex to the Regulation, i.e. products derived from recombinant DNA technology. It results in a Community authorisation applicable in all 15 Member States at the same time, which will soon become a larger Community of 25 Member States after enlargement on 1 May 2004. There is also Part B to the Annex to Council Regulation 2309/93, which lists a number of criteria including new chemical entities, new delivery systems and innovative claims, with which any non-biotechnology product must comply if, at the discretion of the applicant, application should be made for the centralised procedure. It is relevant to point out here that the CVMP has judged that a new serotype for a biological product not authorised before entry into force of the Regulation meets the criteria set out in Part B defined as a new chemical entity.

The second route of authorisation is the mutual recognition procedure, previously referred to as the decentralised procedure, which is controlled in law by the Directive of Council and Parliament 2001/82. This procedure operates for all conventional products and at the discretion of the applicant, those products which might qualify according to Part B of the Annex to Council Regulation 2309/93, but may be where the sponsor chooses not to commercialise his product throughout the Community. The procedure involves the authorisation in one Member State of the EU, which is called the Reference Member State and the recognition of that same authorisation by the remaining Member States called the Concerned Member States. National authorisation may still exist where the sponsor wishes to license it in only one Member State.

It may be useful at this juncture to speak about the spirit of the legislation and to ascertain what the legislator felt was appropriate and what was intended when writing the legislation. In the initial legislation drafted early in the 1980s it would have been difficult for the legislator to foresee what might have been the situation at the beginning of the 21st century, leading to the situation faced today with this availability problem. Therefore I think it is imperative as new legislation is prepared, that the experience of the past is focussed on in some depth. Furthermore it is in the interests of all those involved in providing effective treatment to animals, that representation is made at the highest level by those organisations with access into the Commission and the legislator, for example, the Federation of Veterinarians of Europe and the International Federation of Animal Health, and of course the Member States who have the opportunity through the Council of Ministers to convince the powers-that-be of the need for such medicines.

We should be left in no doubt that the Community sees the primary purpose of the rules for the authorisation and distribution of veterinary medicinal products as being the safeguarding of public health and not necessarily the provision of a duty of care for animal health and welfare. This is why the legislation governing the authorisation of medicines demands that a scientific evaluation of a product must result in assurance of its quality, safety and efficacy, and that concepts of harmfulness and therapeutic efficacy must be examined in considerable depth in relation to one another, to demonstrate a positive benefit-to-risk ratio. Whenever the CVMP adopts a scientific opinion in respect of a new application, which in turn becomes a Community Decision, the assessment reports to the committee are published as European Public Assessment Reports by EMEA. In the EPARs the final section is always dedicated to a risk/benefit analysis of the product in question. In summary, therefore, it is recognised that all medicines may have a risk and that what is being sought is not zero risk. As long as the benefits outweigh such risks, the products could make it to the market place. Specifically for immunologicals, batch consistency of course has to be assured, as well as standards and protocols for the performance tests and trials which must be consistent throughout the EU so that decisions are reached on the basis of uniform tests being applied to uniform criteria or guidelines.

PRACTICAL IMPLEMENTATION OF THE LEGISLATION

Trying to achieve harmonisation between regulators of 15 sovereign Member States has had its difficulties, and certainly this is true in the mutual recognition procedure. Despite having guidelines and position papers, a common approach in a single European market to an assessment of the dossier can prove very difficult. Evidence would suggest that despite the progress made in harmonising the testing requirements of the EU, various experts, when reviewing dossiers, will have their own angle on the data presented and their own interpretation of the guidelines, which can undermine what is meant to be a mutual recognition procedure. It can quite often be difficult to reach agreement between experts assessing the same dossier according to the same legislation and the same guidelines.

EMEA/CVMP APPROACH TO THE MINOR USES MINOR SPECIES PROBLEM

For more than five years, the problem of availability of medicines for minor uses and minor species has been recognised and was highlighted initially by the inability to establish maximum residue limits in the EU for many of the old products after the entry into force of the MRL legislation Council Regulation 2377/90 on 1 January 1992. This Regulation required that any medicinal product intended for veterinary use in food animals had to have a maximum residue limit established for the active substance contained in it. When the EMEA opened in 1995, the responsibility for establishing MRLs for all the old substances on the market on entry into force of the MRL legislation, fell to the CVMP and its Safety Working Party. Not only did the Agency deal with application for new MRLs, but also had to address somewhere between 700-800 old products that needed to have MRLs established.

It was as a result of this exercise that a considerable loss of many old veterinary medicines took place, because the data were not satisfactory to meet the criteria for the requirements in the legislation, or simply some of the companies felt that they did not have the resources, or that the market was not worth the investment necessary to update their dossiers to comply with the legislation.

As a consequence of these difficulties, many of the interested parties at the time, including the industry federation, FEDESA, the Federation of Veterinarians of Europe, the EMEA/CVMP and the Commission came together and hosted a meeting of Interested Parties in July 1999 at the Commission in Brussels. As a result the EMEA created a Task Force, which included representatives from industry, from the veterinarians, from the European Parliament and the Member States, to consider the outcome of the conference and the issues it had highlighted as being in need of resolution. The recommendations of the EMEA Task Force actually formed the basis of many of the recommendations, which the Commission adopted, and published a Communication to Council and Parliament on the Availability of Medicines (Com (2000) 806-final, 5 December 200). One of the first recommendations was to try and address the MRL problem since that had been the initial source of the difficulties, with a call for extrapolation of MRLs established for substances in major species such as cattle, pigs and poultry, to minor species. Initially among regulators, both at the Commission and at the Member State level, there was some scepticism as to the possibilities associated with such extrapolation. There were very firm beliefs that the patterns of metabolism for many of the substances would differ significantly between the species. In the event, this proved not to be the case and an ad hoc group of experts to the CVMP, over a period of two to three years, took an in-depth retrospective look at all the MRLs that had been established in the major species for the major product classes and found, remarkably, that there were many similarities. In particular, many substances seemed to be metabolised in rather similar patterns in the different species with the same marker residue and the same target tissue being prevalent. With that as the basis, there has been a considerable success story in extrapolating some of these major species MRLs to minor species. In addition, the Task Force at the EMEA proposed (and this was taken up in the Commission communication) to consider relaxation of the cascade allowing for exceptional off-label use where medicines were not available to treat certain minor species. However, the application of the particular article in legislation, which allows such off-label use as a default mechanism, had to date been applied in a rather heterogeneous manner throughout the Member States. Nevertheless, where products are not available in that species or, failing that, in any other species and/or in man, reliance on the provisions of the article of the cascade does provide a short-term solution to the provision of such medicines.

The Industry Position

It has become very clear that much of the problem of availability is largely due in part to the problem of cost of research and development being a disincentive to industry to bring such new products to the market when the return on investment is so low: however, the indication from industry colleagues, that selling such products at a reduced margin might make it attractive, is very encouraging. Such an approach needs to be communicated to the Commission, who often use the argument that industry would never participate in such initiatives, without having financial incentives that are provided with the larger mainstream products, to resist providing support to the MUMS policy overall.

Nevertheless, the conventional wisdom now seems to be that for pharmaceuticals there will not be much opportunity to develop novel products for minor species. Every effort should be made to retain those that are already marketed for major species and extend their use to minor species, rather than seek to depend on the possibility of new molecules being developed specifically for these animals. For biologicals, the picture is of course different, with little opportunity to extrapolate vaccine use from one species to another and here it may well be that a guaranteed return on investment with sufficient commercialisation of products having been developed for minor uses and minor species will not be forthcoming. There may be the provision of Community funds to finance research and there may be ways of waiving registration fees, but in order to make the market-place an attractive one for companies to develop biologicals, Member State governments may have to look to state funding to advance product development and entry into the marketplace, and this should certainly be the basis of further discussion.

The CVMP Position Paper on Minor Uses Minor Species Policy

The CVMP adopted this position paper (EMEA/CVMP/477/03-Consultation-corr) for consultation on the availability of minor use and minor species in June 2003, which is a landmark document for the CVMP. The paper attempts to define the problem, giving the background legislative situation in the EU with regard to requirements for authorisation of medicines, and it also attempts to define major and minor species, because to date no legislative definitions exist. The paper describes the activities undertaken so far by the CVMP, as has been discussed earlier in this paper, which sets out a strategic action plan, with short, medium and long-term goals.

It calls for better interpretation of existing legal provisions in respect of provisional marketing authorisations, and explains that the possibility might exist in certain well-defined situations and according to set criteria for authorisation of certain medicines where data are still outstanding and which could be submitted and considered after the initial authorisation agreed to on a provisional basis. A proposal is also made for the possibility of free scientific advice for marketing authorisations and MRL applications for products intended for use in minor uses and minor species. Indeed, at its October 2003 meeting the Management Board of the Agency approved a pilot project for the granting of free scientific advice to companies considering the development of such products with a sum of € 100,000 being set aside for this purpose. Continued efforts will be made to extrapolate major species MRLs to minor ones, and importantly the working parties of the CVMP have been requested to elaborate on the possible reductions in regulatory burdens in reflecting the minimum data requirements for marketing authorisation for products for minor uses and minor species. Clearly such an action plan will also require a harmonised approach from the national regulatory authorities for products for such use in the mutual recognition procedure, and encouragement to achieve this alongside possible fee waivers and fee reductions will be discussed with the Heads of Veterinary Agencies (HEVRA).

In the long-term the strategic action plan calls for a specific legal framework on minor uses and minor species to allow for the designation of such products, the possibility of protocol assistance, market exclusivity (10 years ?), procedural guidance and further Community funding. In addition, it is suggested that the centralised procedure be made compulsory for all such products with adjustments for market introduction in the different countries, depending on animal populations. Some discussion has also been covered on the possibility of Community funding under the Community framework programmes (DG Research) to fund the research and development of such products once the needs are identified according to agreed criteria. On the provision of funds, further discussion should be undertaken with DG Research, which publishes under its framework programme various thematic action areas, and within each thematic action area, it calls for a network of excellence to be put together on the parties that would be interested.

In conclusion, the EMEA/CVMP very much welcomes the opportunity to consult widely on its position paper, and the date for conclusion of the consultation period is 16 December 2003. The Agency wishes to encourage all those parties, particularly those represented here at this conference, to provide as much input as possible in an attempt to reach a consensus on the direction that the CVMP should now be moving in to achieve the goals it wishes to pursue.

Dr. P.G.H Jones, Veterinary Medicines & Inspections, EMEA, 7 Westferry Circus, Canary Wharf, London E14 4HB, United Kingdom.
E-mail: peter.jones@emea.eu.int

Jungbäck C (ed): Consideration of Alternative Licensing Procedures for Vaccines for Minor Species, Minor Indications and Autogenous/Autologous Products.
Dev Biol. Basel, Karger, 2004, vol 117, pp 159-164.

Use of Vaccines for Minor Species – Minor Indications

T. Soós

Control Institute for Veterinary Biologicals and Drugs, Budapest, Hungary

Introduction

It is generally recognised that one of the most significant achievements of medicine in the past two hundred years has been the development and successful application of vaccines. Spectacular examples illustrating the value of vaccination include the eradication of human smallpox and successful prevention of the spread of numerous infectious animal diseases and reduction of the economic losses caused by them.

We can see that the application of new biotechnological and immunological knowledge has opened a new era also in vaccinology: the vaccine manufacturing industry has made great progress, new vaccines have been developed, and the quality, safety and efficacy of vaccines have improved.

Parallel to these developments the requirement system of vaccine authorisation and testing has also changed substantially. In my view, this development is not restricted to the use of up-to-date testing methods (e.g. ELISA, PCR) or the elaboration of detailed regulations setting strict requirements. In my view, the essence of development is that the working philosophy of the regulatory authorities has changed. An authority that strives for performing high-quality work realises that by assisting the industry with its unique means, it serves the interests of public health and animal health. As a result, it will make efforts to solve problems jointly, which is clearly illustrated also by the present conference.

The stricter regulatory requirements, however, have drawbacks as well: the increased R & D costs of products and the higher developmental costs of manufacturing sites are well known, together with the paradoxical phenomenon that, despite the substantial progress of vaccinology as a whole, product shortages may arise in certain fields. The MUMS problem is also such a phenomenon.

Materials and Methods (defining the problem)

How can the essence of the MUMS problem be summarised briefly?

(i) The animal owners' wish to make use of the advantages of vaccination in all animal species is **a rightful demand**. Product shortages should not occur in any field.

(ii) The **demand of the industry** to have its development expenditure recovered and to be able to work with reasonable R & D costs should also be considered a rightful claim. The demand of the industry for clear, unambiguous and consistent regulations that facilitate the marketing of products is also legitimate.

(iii) **The authorities also rightfully lay claim** to a consistent and transparent procedure and to the avoidance of case-by-case decisions. Being able to meet the demands of the market players is a rightful expectation of the authorities, in the interest of their own self-esteem.

In brief, we can say that we must find ways and means to fulfil the above-listed rightful demands in a fair manner, by trying to co-ordinate the scientific and practical aspects during rule-making and by taking into consideration the well-known unique properties and market characteristics of immunobiological products [1,2].

Experience gained in related fields

(i) The significance of MUMS has already been recognised earlier in the field of veterinary medicinal products, and several adequate measures have also been taken. The events that have taken place so far and the special literature of the subject can be regarded as known. However, certain elements of the pharmacological approach can be used as a starting point. Therefore, I consider it my obligation to mention some outstandingly important publications [1-10]. We can state that the most important elements of the European MUMS policy have already been outlined.

(ii) In the field of vaccines for human use some important statements have been made [5], some of which could possibly be used also in the field of vaccines for veterinary use.

The characteristics of immunobiological products and MUMS

When answering questions related to MUMS, the characteristics of immunobiological products must be taken into account. It is known that while the risk of medicines is product-specific, that of vaccines can be said to be batch-specific. A further important difference between the two product groups is the purpose of application (therapeutic and preventive, respectively) and the significance in disease control; therefore, it is of fundamental importance to ensure the safety and efficacy of vaccines and to take into consideration the epizootiological aspects.

Results and Discussion

The IWP has discussed the vaccine characteristics related to the applicability of the EWP principles on the basis of the valuable comments made by C. Jungbäck [11,12] and M. Ilott [13]. Subsequently, the EMEA/CVMP has drafted the position paper that can be regarded as a guideline [9]. Hopefully it is not a futile attempt to try to find further answers to the questions that arise.

Defining minor species

The following questions must be answered:

(i) Can the approach of the EWP, i.e. classification on the basis of the population size of the different animal species, be applied? If not, are statistical surveys necessary?

(ii) In the EU consisting of 25 states, can MS be defined also in relation to immunobiological products? Alternatively, taking into consideration the inter-country differences in animal breeding or in the epizootiological importance of specific infectious diseases, would it be expedient to define only general principles that would make reclassification between minor and major species possible for the member states in a flexible manner?

In my view, at present it would be expedient to leave off the time-consuming and costly statistical surveys and to use the definition made by EMEA/CVMP [minor species can be defined as animals other than cattle (dairy and meat animals), sheep (meat animals), pigs, chickens (including laying hens), dogs, cats and *Salmonidae*].

In addition to the consistent application of the EU definition, disease control arguments could be brought up in support of the practice that, whenever this is justified, some member states should regard as major species certain animal species classified as minor species. A drawback of this aspiration to a flexible procedure is, however, that during the MRP procedures serious consultation difficulties may occur; therefore, decisions should be preceded by very thorough consideration.

Defining the minor indication

It is known that the EWP 'has proposed a threshold for minor indication based on sales value. A figure of approximately two million Euros for total European sales would be a reasonable point for consultation with industry'. The opinion of vaccinologists is not uniform; according to some specialists 'for immunologicals a similar approach would be both consistent and logical' [13], while other experts raise the question 'how far can we follow these quantifications with respect for IVMPs' [11,12].

According to the EMEA/CVMP [9], 'the only practical approach at present seems to identify a minor use on a case-by-case... because of the difficulties in obtaining any useful data'.... 'The minor use approvals should only be considered by one single expert body. Once experience had been gained criteria could be defined.'

At present this proposal seems to be the most reasonable solution; however, efforts should be made to establish a uniform and consistent procedure as soon as possible; therefore, it would be valuable to find answers also to further questions that may arise.

(i) Isn't the threshold of two million Euros to high? In the absence of exact sales data I can only set forth my personal opinion: it does seem to be high. It would be expedient to determine the threshold during consultations with the industry.

(ii) How do we wish to handle the annual changes of sales data? As a result of facilitated marketing relating to minor use, the sales value can possibly exceed the threshold rapidly, in which case the mitigated requirement will not be applicable in the subsequent year. It is to be hoped that the introduction of the system of conditional authorisations valid for two to three years will also give an answer to that question. During the term of validity of the authorisation the industry would be able to make preparations for fulfilling the entire system of requirements, should this possibly be necessary.

(iii) It requires consideration whether classification as a minor indication can be done exclusively on the basis of sales criteria. It would be reasonable to take into account the epizootiological and public health aspects (e.g. OIE 'A' list; zoonoses).

In my opinion, on the basis of the current sales values it would be paradoxical to regard vaccines against foot-and-mouth disease (FMD) and classical swine fever (CSF) as 'minor use' cases and to ease the requirements relating to them. What is the situation with vaccines against zoonoses? Let us take as an example the oral vaccine serving for immunisation of foxes against rabies. It follows from the definition that the fox should be regarded as a minor species; however, you will probably agree with me in that it would be difficult to imagine a facilitation in the requirement system in this case due to the necessity of fighting off sylvatic rabies and because of the special method of application of the vaccine.

I think these two examples prove that at present it would be difficult to propose a definition better than the case-by-case definition recommended by the CVMP, however much we would like to do that. However, I would consider it expedient and propose it for consideration that the MUMS affairs relating to immunobiological products should remain within the competence of the Immunological Working Party (IWP), even if an Orphan Veterinary Medicinal Products Working Party were to be set up.

Immunobiological products against what diseases can be classified as 'minor use'?

During the earlier technical discussions several infectious diseases have been mentioned, the immunobiological products against which can be assigned to this category with the specialists' approval (Anthrax, Botulism, Equine viral arteritis, Equine coronavirus, Japanese encephalitis, Louping ill, Q fever). Furthermore, the sheep disease caused by *C. septicum* (bradsot), the diseases caused by certain *Haemophilus* species (*H. somnus, H. parasuis*) and those due to *Campylobacter fetus* subspecies *fetus* should also be considered for potential classification into this category. Probably the vaccines against duck virus hepatitis and duck virus enteritis also fit into this category. The cases falling within the scope of line extension are also beginning to take shape [extension of bovine vaccines to goats, deer, buffaloes; extension of chicken vaccines to ducks, geese (and possibly to turkeys), extension of vaccines against bovine/avian salmonellosis to pigs; extension of vaccines against bovine leptospirosis to pigs].

I do not think that it would be my task to present a complete list of diseases and I do not even feel myself competent to do so; such a list will obviously be drawn up during further consultations.

Requirements

Authorisation procedure

Rendering possible all three procedures (Centralised, MRP and National) seems to be a useful and rational approach. Permitting the central procedure based on payment of a fair charge may exert a stimulating effect on the R & D sector and facilitate harmonisation of the scientific and the practical aspects. This would also be useful because vaccines developed by the use of the rDNS technique could markedly facilitate the solution of MUMS problems.

The conditional authorisation

It is to be hoped that the introduction of the conditional (and temporary) authorisation would greatly facilitate the management of MUMS matters.

(i) As set forth above, this conditional authorisation would regulate the sales value limits determined for the 'minor use' category on the basis of accurately specified time spans.

(ii) It would render possible the faster marketing of products, as certain requirements of the documents would have to be fulfilled only during the time of conditional marketing (see below).

(iii) The faster marketing of products and the marketing of a larger number of products could also facilitate the preparation of European Pharmacopoeia monographs.

Requirements of dossiers

I propose the following facilitated parts for discussion:

Part II

Facilitation in Part II, Chapter F: Depending on product type, the conditional authorisation could be issued if the results of the four- to six-month real-time stability tests conformed to the requirements. Further stability data could be compiled by applicant during the time of marketing on the basis of conditional authorisation. By the regular submission of a Periodic Stability Report (PSR) a prolongation could be made even during the validity of the conditional authorisation.

Line extension: An alternative approach is possible: (i) as the dossiers prepared for major species/major use must be available, the industry will surely be able to submit the full documentation; (ii) by permitting the submission of the shortened Part II dossier with reference to the original full dossier, administrative work (and in the case of national procedures, possibly translation costs) could be saved.

Part III

In the case of **live vaccines** a facilitation may presumably be allowed only in the immune status of animals used for safety tests: (i) in the case of extension of avian vaccines, experiments on SPF animals can be omitted; (ii) in the case of other products, experiments performed on animals of 'non-vaccinated' immune status are acceptable. In the case of **inactivated vaccines** laboratory experiments performed with a single dose on non-vaccinated animals and pilot-scale or reduced plant-scale experiments seem to be sufficient.

The issue of the conditional and temporary authorisation could be combined with the obligation to monitor the practical application of the product and to report the results of that monitoring (some kind of PSUR of elevated level).

Part IV

Depending on the 'nature of protection' specified in the indications of the vaccine there may be differences in the efficacy requirements, but 'the development of an immunological parameter, such as a serological response' seems to be acceptable. Similarly, as in the previous point, drafting of a Periodic Efficacy Update Report (PEUR) and Periodic Report on the Duration of Immunity would be worth considering so that the knowledge relating to the given product could be expanded by the time of expiry of the conditional authorisation.

REFERENCES

1. Clayton R, Zänker S: Availability of Veterinary Medicinal Products. Regulatory Affairs Journal 1999; 10: 956-958.
2 Clayton R, Zänker S: Towards an EU policy for Veterinary Medicinal Products for Minor Use, Minor Species, Part 1. Regulatory Affairs Journal 2002; 13 (6): 499-504.
3 Clayton R, Zänker S: Towards an EU policy for Veterinary Medicinal Products for Minor Use, Minor Species, Part 2. Regulatory Affairs Journal 2002; 13 (7): 579-584.
4 Clayton R, Zänker S: Towards an EU policy for Veterinary Medicinal Products for Minor Use, Minor Species, Part 3. Regulatory Affairs Journal 2002; 13 (8): 661-667.
5 Brown F, Gust I (eds): Orphan Vaccines-Bridging the Gap. Development in Biologicals, Basel, Karger, 2002, vol 110.
6 Guest G: Antimicrobials and minor species/minor indications. 5th International Technical Consultation on Veterinary Drug Registration, The Hague, 1990.
7 Owusu J: Minor animal species and therapeutic claims, flexible labelling use in Australia. 7th International Technical Consultation on Veterinary Drug Registration, Paris, 1994.
8 EMEA/CVMP/610/01-Consultation: Points to consider regarding efficacy requirements for minor species and minor indications.
9 EMEA/CVMP/477/03-consultation: position paper regarding availability of products for minor uses and minor species (MUMS).
10 Communication from the Commission to the Council and the European Parliament 5/12/200-COM (2000) 806.final-on "Availability of veterinary medicinal products".
11 CVMP/IWP/59/02 Position paper on Use of Vaccines for Minor Species-Minor Indications (work with EWP); Comments from C. Jungbäck on the Points to consider regarding efficacy requirements for minor species-minor indications.
12 CVMP/IWP/32/03 Position paper on Use of Vaccines for Minor Species-Minor Indications (work with EWP); Comments from C. Jungbäck on the Points to consider regarding efficacy requirements for minor species-minor indications.
13 CVMP/IWP/49/03 Position paper on Use of Vaccines for Minor Species-Minor Indications (work with EWP); Comments from M. Ilott on the Points to consider regarding efficacy requirements for minor species-minor indications.

Prof. T. Soós, Control Institute for Veterinary Biologicals and Drugs, X. Szállás u.8, H-1107 Budapest, Hungary.
E-mail: soost@oai.hu

Jungbäck C (ed): Consideration of Alternative Licensing Procedures for Vaccines for Minor Species, Minor Indications and Autogenous/Autologous Products.
Dev Biol. Basel, Karger, 2004, vol 117, pp 165-170.

Vaccines for Minor Species and Minor Indications: Current Situation and Concepts in Germany – Feasible Approaches for the Future – Authorities' View –

E. Werner

Paul-Ehrlich-Institut, Langen, Germany

Abstract: About 350 immunological products for veterinary use are authorised for different species and indications in Germany. Vaccines licensed for minor species and minor indications are very rare. Existing products are being withdrawn from the market if the limited market size does not justify any investment for production and marketing, as well as to update the dossiers in accordance with the current regulatory requirements if normally only a limited data set regarding safety and efficacy of the products is available. Subsequently an increase of off-label use of authorised products and of autologous or of non-licensed immunological products are observed. The issue of availability of veterinary immunological medicines in minor species and minor indications has been recognised as a problem in the past few years. A brief review of the current legal situation in Germany and current examples are presented.

It is therefore necessary to establish the standards of quality, safety and efficacy for veterinary immunological products intended for minor species and minor indications. There is a need to define a harmonised procedure to authorise products for minor species and minor indications on the basis of agreed minimum requirements. Feasible approaches for revision of requirements for the registration of vaccines for minor species and minor indications are proposed.

INTRODUCTION

The problem of the availability of veterinary immunological products for minor uses/indications and minor species (MUMS) has been discussed for a considerable time worldwide. The availability problem is not a specific issue for the European Union. Due to globalisation the relative importance of minor species has become less. In addition the introduction and implementation of the harmonised pharmaceutical legislation in the European Union have led to a reduction in the range of vaccines and other immunological products available on the market. Over the past few years an application assessment process has been established with respect to the quality, safety and efficacy of vaccines. The vaccine approval model works well for products for animals defined as major species. However, it does not work satisfactorily with vaccines for other animal species, the so-called "minor" species. The limited market for vaccines intended for minor species or for minor use and the subsequent unprofitable use are reasons for the failure of this model. There are often insufficient economic incentives to motivate companies to develop the data necessary to support approvals. Consequently, manufacturers have not, in many cases, been willing to fund research to obtain these data. The manufacturer is no longer in a position to recoup the costs of developing vaccines for MUMS and to obtain marketing authorisations for MUMS products. Accordingly, only a small number of vaccines intended for minor species or for minor uses have been authorised and are legally marketed at the present time. Therefore, there is a critical shortage of approved animal MUMS vaccines. Because of the limited availability of MUMS products, veterinarians, animal owners, and livestock producers may have only restricted options for the use of prophylactic measures such as vaccinations of these animals against a multitude of diseases. In many cases, the choices available are to leave the animals unvaccinated or to vaccinate the animal with an unauthorised product. The shortage of approved vaccines results in animal suffering, lost of animal life, and financial loss to those who raise the animals. But humans have a responsibility to try to prevent the suffering and death that is caused by the shortage of authorised vaccines for the care of such animals. Furthermore, the absence of vaccination may lead to increased public health and environment hazards.

Based on the analysis of the current situation regarding the legislation in force, of the need of vaccines for minor species/minor use and of available options for the use of MUMS products in different countries, necessary and possible changes in the actual legal provisions shall be discussed with the objectives of simplifying procedures for the registration of MUMS products, to define criteria for safety and efficacy testing as well as to identify diseases belong to this area. Proposals should be developed which clearly indicate the quality, safety and efficacy data requirements for MUMS vaccines and identify a harmonised procedure to authorise these products on the basis of an agreed minimum data package.

Basic Principles of a Minor Species and Minor Use Policy

The analysis of the current situation has shown that precise and standardised criteria for the definition of minor species or minor use do not exist. No harmonised, clearly defined procedures for the authorisation of MUMS vaccines, are available. In a few countries, specific authorisation procedures for MUMS products are in place, e.g. provisional authorisations may be granted for a limited time.

The CVMP Position Paper (EMEA/CVMP/477/03) regarding the availability of products for minor uses and minor species states: "The goal of the CVMP is to establish the standards of quality, safety and efficacy for veterinary medicinal products for medicines intended for minor uses and minor species, both for pharmaceutical and immunological products."

The first criteria for the definition of a species as a major or a minor species are proposed in this position paper. The number of animals on the European Union market should be the basis for classification. Other factors, such as the low economic value of the single animal or the appropriate animal product, should be taken into consideration. For mammalian species a threshold value of 15 million animals, for poultry a threshold value of 200 million and for fish a threshold value of 100,000 tons should be fulfilled. Two exemptions are allowed. About 20 million dairy sheep exist in the European Union. But if they have a very low milk yield compared to dairy cattle they should not be defined as a major species. If the single animal has a low financial value in meat and fur-producing, such as rabbits, they are defined as minor species although about 260 million animals exist in the European Union.

As a result the following species are defined as major: cattle (dairy and meat animals), sheep (meat animals), pigs, chickens (including laying hens), salmonidae, dogs and cats. Therefore all other species are defined as minor species, including horses, turkeys and other avian species, rabbits, goats, as well as mink, ferret, fox, zoo animals, other fishes and honey bees. In the United States of America horses and turkeys are defined as major species. The variation of animal numbers within the Member States of the European Union is not taken into account. But differences between the single Member States regarding the assessment of a species as major or minor are known. In France turkeys will be classified as major, in Greece goats play an important role. In generally it should be discussed if horses, turkeys and rabbits or some other species are really minor species.

'Minor use' could be a minor indication in a major species for an indication that occurs infrequently or in limited geographical areas, but also for the use of vaccines in minor species. Criteria for classification as minor indications/minor use are not defined. Therefore it is very difficult to establish thresholds for these kinds of vaccines. Applications are normally treated and assessed on a case-by-case basis.

Current Situation in Germany

In Germany about 30% of the veterinary medicinal product used in the veterinary practice are vaccines and sera. Over 350 veterinary immunological products are registered for different target species and indications. A marketing authorisation exists for about 45 products for cattle, 70 for pigs, 110 for poultry, including chicken, turkey, duck, goose, pigeon and canary, six for sheep, 30 for horses, 55 for dogs, 30 for cats, 10 for rabbits as well as single products for fish, fox, and mink.

Examples for minor indications are the following from the German point of view:

- Paratuberculosis in cattle, sheep, goats, other ruminants and zoo animals (some years ago a vaccine was available for use in cattle).
- Q fever in cattle (some years ago a vaccine was available for use in cattle).
- Chlamydia infection in cattle and sheep (one live vaccine is available for sheep, except pregnant animals).

- Botulismus in cattle, horses and aquatic birds such as swans, ducks, geese (in exceptional cases a vaccine is imported from South Africa).
- Rabies and distemper in minks and ferrets, arctic fox, marten, seals, otters, panda.
- Orthopoxvirus infection in elephants, rhinoceros, tapir.
- Equine viral arteritis in horses
- Contagious ecthyma in sheep
- Newcastle disease in ducks, geese, pheasants, quails
- Canary pox infection
- Coccidiosis in turkeys
- Mycosis in rabbits and guinea pigs

For the immunisation against a few of the above-mentioned diseases vaccines were authorised for the German market in the past; however in the meantime most of them have been withdrawn. The causes were the limited market size as well as the availability of only a limited data set regarding safety and efficacy to update the dossier in the vaccine review. The consequence was the loss of MUMS vaccines.

Against further diseases vaccines are developed by different companies, but Marketing Authorisation is not applied for if e.g. no batch potency test is available or if it is difficult to demonstrate the efficacy in the target species by a challenge model or by serological testing. In single cases, the appropriate veterinary vaccines are imported from another country under strict conditions for a clearly defined use.

In practice, authorised products are being used off-label, e.g. vaccines for cattle or sheep are used in goats, vaccines for chickens in turkeys and ducks, or autologous vaccines are prepared and administered.

Concepts and Feasible Approaches for the Future

The harmonised European legislation for immunological products includes no exemptions concerning the requirements for quality, safety and efficacy of MUMS vaccines. However, the need to modify the current legislation in relation to MUMS vaccines and to make the development of these products more attractive have already been identified. Special items for this group of vaccines have not yet been defined. Measures should include a reduced data package, simplified harmonised registration and maintenance procedures, a reasonable approach regarding fee structures, reduced administrative burden, acceptance of data from third parties, international packaging and SPC lay-out to reduce the number of languages.

The objectives of these measures are shorter development times for MUMS vaccines and a quicker response to disease threat.

In principle, all three authorisation procedures (the centralised, the mutual recognition and the national authorisation procedure) should be conducted to obtain a marketing authorisation for a MUMS product. But, depending on the product, other authorisation procedures should be applicable for these products. Options are provisional or conditional licences as well as line extensions and variations.

Different categories of applications for MUMS are conceivable:

- the use of a veterinary vaccine authorised for a major species in a minor species;
- the use of an authorised veterinary vaccine for a minor use;
- the use of an entirely new veterinary vaccine in a minor species or for a minor indication;
- the use of an available human vaccine in a minor species or for a minor indication.

The formulation of the data requirements regarding quality, safety and efficacy for MUMS vaccines should be considered in the context of both the use of already existing vaccines and new vaccine development only for MUMS.

In the case of an existing product a satisfactory set of supporting quality data are already available for this vaccine. A full part II dossier could be supplied in support of an application. However, a shortened documentation with reference to the original dossier appears adequate. It should be possible to update the export reports by an addendum in a reduced number of languages. Regarding safety data it should be discussed to what extent extrapolation is possible to the new species or new indication. For live vaccines it should be considered whether a full safety package regarding the special requirements such as reversion to virulence, spread of the vaccine strain, dissemination etc. are necessary.

In the case of a new product for MUMS, a full supporting quality data package will normally be required. Depending on the active substances, the dosage etc., the data requirements might be reduced for specific areas. Production validation should be performed with pilot batches. For active substance analysis and stability as well as for final product batch analysis and stability, data would be required for two pilot batches only. Data for production batches should be submitted when available. For the evaluation of safety and efficacy the same trials should be included. In these studies representative batches instead of minimum or maximum batches should be used. Whenever possible, efficacy should be demonstrated by serology.

For MUMS products there will be a need for an efficient follow-up and vaccino-vigilance which has to be associated with a more flexible approach and less stringent requirements.

Conclusions

The limited availability or the lack of vaccines for minor species and minor use pose a threat not only for the appropriate animal species but also for other animal species, for human health and for the environment. Therefore it is necessary to find a more pragmatic approach to the evaluation of the quality, safety and efficacy of MUMS vaccines. A detailed and reasonable risk-benefit assessment should be provided, taking into consideration the importance and influence of the specific disease for animal welfare, human health and environment.

References

1 EMEA/CVMP/477/03. Position paper regarding the availability of products for minor uses and minor species (MUMS).

Dr. E. Werner, Paul-Ehrlich-Institut, Paul-Ehrlich-Str. 51-59, D-63225 Langen, Germany.
E-mail: weres@pei.de

List of Participants

AERTS Rene M.L., Intervet International B.V., Wim de Körverstraat 35, P.O. Box 31, NL-5830 Boxmeer, The Netherlands.

AKERBLOM Lennart, MPA Sweden, P.O. Box 26, S-751 03 Uppsala, Sweden.

BEHR Klaus-Peter, Heidemark GmbH, Mülenstrasse 13, D-49685 Höltinghausen, Germany.

BIESSMANN Albrecht, Lohmann Animal Health GmbH & Co, Heinz-Lohmann-Strasse 4, D-27472 Cuxhaven, Germany.

BÖNISCH Brigitte, Merial S.A.S., 29, av. Tony Garnier, F-69007 Lyon, France.

BROWN Karen, Dermal Research Laboratories, Inc., 5501 NW Foxhill Road, Parkville, MO 64152, USA.

BUECHNER Jutta, Streetzer Weg 15a, D-06862 Rodleben, Germany.

BURES Jiri, Institute for the State Control of Veterinary Biologicals and Medicaments, Hudcova 56a, Brno 62100, Czech Republic.

CARLSON Madonna M., Fort Dodge Animal Health, 800 Fifth Street N.W., P.O. Box 518, Fort Dodge, IA 50501, USA.

CHAPEK Mary Lou, MVP Laboratories, Inc., 5404 Miller Avenue, Ralston, NE 68127, USA.

CHASE Christopher, Department of Veterinary Science, South Dakota State University, P.O. Box 2175, ADR Rm 125, Brookings, SD 57007, USA.

CHATON-SCHAFFNER Mireille, Ceva Santé Animale, Z.I. La Ballastière, F-33500 Libourne, France.

DE FOUCAULD Jean, CEVA-Phylaxia, Szállás u.5, H-1107 Budapest, Hungary.

DRAAYER Hans, Pfizer Animal Health, 0225-190-43, 5300 N. 28th Street, Richland, MI 49083. USA.

ELBERS Knut, Boehringer Ingelheim Vetmedica GmbH, Gr. Biological R & D, D-55435 Ingelheim, Germany.

EMANUELE Maria Chiara, Ist. Zooprofilattico Sperimentale della Sicilia, Via G. Marinuzzi 3, I-90129 Palermo, Italy.

ESPESETH David, IABs, 404 Long Leaf Drive, Perkasie, PA 18944, USA.

FIGA Marta, Laboratorios Hipra S.A., Av. La Selva 135, ES-17170 Amer (Girona), Spain.

FORBRIG Thomas, Dr. Felgenträger & Co., Oeko-chem. und Pharma GmbH, Zerbster Str. 7a, D-06862 Rodleben, Germany.

GAUDRY Daniel, 46 Inlets Blvd, Nokomis, FL 34275, USA.

GRAVENDYCK Marcus, Intervet International BV, Wim de Körverstraat 35, P.O. Box 31, NL-5830 AA Boxmeer, The Netherlands.

GUTIERREZ TEJERINA José, Laboratorios Calier, S.A., C/Alta Ribagorza 6-8, Mas Blau II, ES-08820 El Prat de Llobregat (Barcelona), Spain.

HILL Richard E., Center for Veterinary Biologicals(CVB), USDA, APHIS, Veterinary Services, 510 South 17th Street, Suite 104, Ames, IA 50010, USA.

HOOG Alex, MVP Laboratories, Inc., 5404 Miller Ave, Ralston, NE 68127, USA.

HUFF Joseph, Colorado Serum Company, 4950 York Street, Denver, CO 80216-0428, USA.

ILOTT Martin, Veterinary Medicines Directorate (VMD), Woodham Lane, New Haw, Addlestone, Surrey KT15 3LS, United Kingdom.

JAKAVA-VILJANEN Miia, Nat. Vet. And Food Res. Inst., EELA, P.O. Box 45, Hämaentie 57, FI-00581 Helsinki, Finland.

JONES Peter, European Agency for the Evaluation of Medicinal Products (EMEA), 7 Westferry Circus, Canary Wharf, London E14 4HB, U.K.

JUNGBÄCK Carmen, Paul-Ehrlich-Institut, Bundesamt für Sera und Impfstoffe, Paul-Ehrlich-Str. 51-59, D-63225 Langen, Germany.

KOEHLER Bernd, Landesamt für Verbraucherschutz und Landwirtschaft, D-14478 Potsdam, Germany.

KOEHLER Dagmar, Ripac-Labor, D-14478 Potsdam, Germany.

KRIZ Nikolaus, EMEA / EU, 7, Westferry Circus, Canary Wharf, London E14 4HB, U.K.

LANGE Stephan, Boehringer Ingelheim Vetmedica GmbH, D-55216 Ingelheim, Germany.

LEHMANN Kristina, National Agency for Medicines, Mannerheimintie 166, P.O. Box 55, FIN-00301 Helsinki, Finland.

LEMBECK Johannes, LAH Cuxhaven, Herbert-Meyer-Str. 25, D-29556 Suderburg, Germany.

LYSVAG Camilla, Norwegian Medicines Agency, Sven Oftedals vei 6, N-0950 Oslo, Norway.

MACKAY David K.J., Institute for Animal Health, Pirbright Laboratory, Ash Road, Pirbright, Woking, Surrey GU24 0NF, United Kingdom.

MARCA Joan, Laboratorios Calier, S.A., C/Alta Ribagorza 6-8, Mas Blau II, E-08820 El Prat de Llobregat (Barcelona), Spain.

MEINEKE Dietmar, Labor Dr. Thrull, Im Raum 8, D-22946 Trittan, Germany.

MIDTLYNG Paul J., Veso, P.O. Box 8109 DEP, N-0032 Oslo, Norway.

MIRAS Christine, AFSSA - Agence Nationale du Médicament Vétérinaire, La Haute Marche, B.P. 203 Javené, F-35302 Fougères, France.

MOORE Gareth A., (CPAC/ American Veterinary Medicinal Association), 159 Liberty Lane, Pembroke, VA 24136-3078, USA.

MORENO Miguel, Depto Sanidad Animal Fac. Vet. UCM, Anda Puerta de Hierro S/N, E-28040 Madrid, Spain.

MUELLER Kirsten, LVL Lebensmittel-u. Veterinäruntersuchgslabor GmbH, Ecopark Allee 6, D-49685 Emstek, Germany.

NEUBERT Andreas, Impfstoffwerk Dessau-Tornau GmbH, Postfach 400214, D-06855 Roßlau, Germany.

NOLTE Oliver, Hygiene-Institute, Dept of Hygiene & Med Microbiology, Im Neuenheimer Feld 324, D-69120 Heidelberg, Germany.

OTHMAR Brigitte, Lohmann Animal Health GmbH, Heinz-Lohmann-Strasse 4, D-27472 Cuxhaven, Germany.

OTTIGER Hans-Peter, Institut für Viruskrankheiten + Immunoproph., Sensemattstr. 293, CH-3147 Mittelhäusern, Switzerland.

PAPADOPOULOS Orestis, Aristotle University of Thessaloniki (AUTH), Faculty of Veterinary Med., Dept. of Microb. & Infectious Dis., GR-54124 Thessaloniki, Greece.

PAPE Iska, Niedersächsisches Ministerium für den ländlichen Raum, Ernährung, Landwirtschaft und Verbr., Postfach 243, D-30002 Hannover, Germany.

POCHODYLA Andrzej, Vepharm, Ul. Karpinskiego 7, PL-24-100 Polawy, Poland.

REITAN Liv Jorun, National Veterinary Institute, P.O. Box 8156 Dep., N-0033 Oslo, Norway.

ROUMIANTZEFF Micha, 1, rue Dangon, F-69004 Lyon, France.

SCHNEIDER Thomas, German Federal Ministry for Consumer Protection, Food and Agriculture, Rockusstrasse 1, D-53123 Bonn, Germany.

SIEVERDING Erwin, Tierärztliche Praxis am Bergweg, Bergweg 20, D-49393 Lohne, Germany.

SIGGE Claudia, Bundesverband für Tiergesundheit e.V., Aennchenplatz 6, D-53173 Bonn NRW, Germany.

SMITH John A., Fieldale Farms Corp., P.O. Box 558, Baldwin, GA 30511, USA.

SOÓS Tibor, Control Institute for Veterinary Biologicals and Drugs, X. Szállás u.8, H-1107 Budapest, Hungary.

STANGL Elisabeth, Fort Dodge Veterinär GmbH, Adenauerstrasse 20, D-52146 Würselen, Germany.

TELLEZ Sonia, Depto Sanidad Animal Fac. Vet. UCM, Anda Puerta de Hierro S/N, ES-28040 Madrid, Spain.

THIBAULT Eric, Biovac, Angers Technopôle, 4, rue Olivier de Serres, F-49071 Beaucouze Cedex, France.

THIELE Susanne, Intervet International BV, Wim de Körverstraat 35, P O Box 31, NL-5830 AA Boxmeer, The Netherlands.

THRULL Ralf, Medica Lab., Lise-Meitner-Str. 21, D-25524 Itzehoe, Germany.

TOLLIS Maria, Laboratorio di Medicina Veterinaria, Istituto Superiore di Sanità, viale Regina Elena 299, I-00161 Roma, Italy.

VAN DER MAREL Pieter, Intervet International BV, Wim de Körverstraat 35, P O Box 31, NL-5830 AA Boxmeer, The Netherlands.

VAN DER VALK Pieter, Fort Dodge Veterinär GmbH, Adenauerstrasse 20, D-52146 Würselen, Germany.

VANDAELE Bill, BVD Consultants SA, 371, Rue Rolleghem, B-7700 Mouscron, Belgium.

VANNIER Philippe, AFSSA Ploufragan, Zoopole Les Croix, BP 53, F-22440 Ploufragan, France.

VON FREYBURG Martina, Boehringer Ingelheim Vetmedica GmbH, Gr. Biological R & D, D-55435 Ingelheim, Germany.

VOSS Matthias, Lohmann Tierzucht GmbH, Veterinary Laboratory, Abschnede 64, D-27472 Cuxhaven, Germany.

WERNER Esther, Paul-Ehrlich-Institut, Bundesamt für Sera und Impfstoffe, Paul-Ehrlich-Str. 51-59, D-63225 Langen, Germany.

ZÄNKER Susanne, IFAH-Europe, (Int. Federation for Animal Health), 1, rue Defacqz, B-1000 Brussels, Belgium.

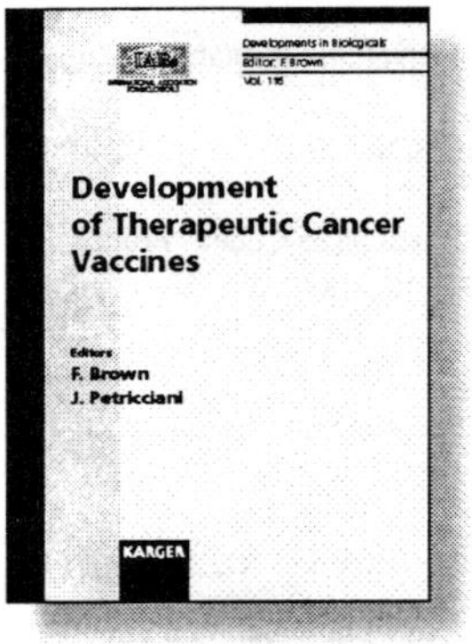
Development
of Therapeutic Cancer
Vaccines
Editors
F. Brown
J. Petricciani
KARGER

Index of Authors

Symposia Series in Immunobiological Standardization

Vol. 1: Talloires 1965	Rabies
Vol. 2: Munich 1965	Neurovirulence of viral vaccines
Vol. 3: Stockholm 1965	Biotechnical developments in bacterial vaccine production
Vol. 4: Royaumont 1965	Immunological methods of biological standardization
Vol. 5: London 1966	Laboratory animals
Vol. 6: Utrecht 1966	Adjuvants of immunity
Vol. 7: Marburg/L. 1967	Assay of combined antigens
Vol. 8: Lyon 1967	Foot-and-Mouth Disease: Variants and immunity
Vol. 9: Paris 1967	Pseudotuberculosis
Vol. 10: London 1967	Biological assay methods of vaccine and sera
22nd Symp., London 1968	Standardization of immunofluorescence. Ed. Blackwell
Vol. 11: London 1968	Rubella vaccines
Vol. 12: Tunis 1968	Brucellosis. Standardization and control of vaccines and reagents
Vol. 13: Utrecht 1969	Pertussis vaccine
Vol. 14: London 1969	Standardization of interferon and interferon inducers
Vol. 15: Berne 1969	Enterobacterial vaccines
Vol. 16: Versailles 1970	Anti-lymphocytic serum
29th Symp., Brighton 1969	Hazards of handling simians. Ed. Lab. Animals Ltd. (4)
Vol. 17: Frankfurt 1970	BCG vaccine
Vol. 18: Copenhagen 1972	HL-A reagents
Vol. 19: Utrecht 1972	Smallpox vaccines
Vol. 20: London 1972	Influenza
Vol. 21: Lyon 1972	Rabies II
Vol. 22: Monaco 1973	The use of vaccines

Developments in Biological Standardization

Vol. 23: Madrid 1973	Sterilization and sterility testing of biological substances
Vol. 24: San Francisco 1973	Preservatives in biological products
Vol. 25: Lyon 1973	Requirements for poultry virus vaccines
Vol. 26: Budapest 1973	Selected veterinary vaccines
Vol. 27: Budapest 1973	Purity of human plasma proteins
Vol. 28: London 1974	Immunity to infections of the respiratory system in man and animals

46th Symp., London 1974	Breeding of simians and their uses in developmental biology. Ed. Lab. Animals Ltd. (6)
Vol. 29: Geneva 1974 (WHO/IABS)	Standardization and control of allergens administered to man
Vol. 30: Milan 1974	Viral hepatitis
Vol. 31: Rabat 1975	Brucellosis (II)
Vol. 32: Paris 1975 (OIE/IABS)	Colstridial sera and vaccines for veterinary use
Vol. 33: Douglas 1975	Vaccination by the non-parenteral route
Vol. 34: Budapest 1976	Pyrogenicity, innocuity and toxicity test systems for biological products
Vol. 35: Lyon 1976	Foot-and-mouth disease vaccines
Vol. 36: Lyon Washington D.C. 1976	Freeze-drying of biological products
Vol. 37: Geneva 1976	Standardization of cell substrates for the production of virus vaccines
Vol. 38: London 1977	Biological preparations in the treatment of cancer
Vol. 39: Geneva 1977	Influenza immunization (II)
Vol. 40: Marburg 1977	Standardization of rabies vaccines (III) (WHO/IABS)
Vol. 41: Guadeloupe 1978	Vaccinations in the developing countries
Vol. 42: Paris 1978	Second General Meeting of European Society of Animal Cell Technology
Vol. 43: Brussels 1978	Immunization: Benefit versus risk factors
Vol. 44: Villars 1979	Test methods for the quality control of plasma proteins
Vol. 45: San Antonio 1979	The Standardization of animals to improve biomedical research, production and control
Vol. 46: Oxford 1979	Third General Meeting of European Society of Animal Cell Technology
Vol. 47: Bilthoven 1980	Reassessment of inactivated poliomyelitis vaccine
Vol. 48: Geneva 1980	Standardization of albumin, plasma substitutes and plasmapheresis
Vol. 49: Leetown 1981	Fish biologics: Serodiagnostics and vaccines
Vol. 50: Heidelberg 1981	Joint ESACT-IABS Meeting on the use of heteroploid and other cell substrates for the production of biologicals
Vol. 51: Lyon 1981	Immunization of adult birds with inactivated oil adjuvant vaccines
Vol. 52: Lyon 1981	Herpes virus of man and animal: Standardization of immunological procedures
Vol. 53: Dublin 1982	Enteric infections in man and animals: Standardization of immunological procedures
Vol. 54: Athens 1982	Viral hepatitis: Standardization in immunoprophylaxis of infections by hepatitis viruses
Vol. 55: Copenhagen 1982	Fifth General Meeting of European Society of Animal Cell Technology
Vol. 56: Algeria 1983	IIIrd International Symposium on Brucellosis
Vol. 57: Paris 1983	Monoclonal antibodies: Standardization of their characterization and use
Vol. 58: Budapest 1983	BCG vaccines and tuberculins
Vol. 59: Geneva 1983	Standardization and control of biologicals produced by recombinant DNA technology
Vol. 60: Gardone Riviera 1983	Production and exploitation of existing and new animal cell substrates
Vol. 61: Geneva 1984	Proceedings of the Fourth International Symposium on pertussis
Vol. 62: Stockholm 1985	Diagnostics and vaccines for parasitic diseases
Vol. 63: San Francisco 1985	Use and standardization of chemically defined antigens
Vol. 64: London 1985	Reduction of animal usage in the development and control of biological products
Vol. 65: Amsterdam 1985	Use and standardization of combined vaccines
Vol. 66: Baden 1985	Advances in animal cell technology: cell engineering, evaluation and exploitation

Vol. 67: Melbourne 1986	Standardization in blood fractionation including coagulation factors
Vol. 68: Geneva 1986	Cells – Products – Safety
Vol. 69: London 1987	Cytokines: Laboratory and clinical evaluation
Vol. 70: Arlington, 1988	Continuous cell lines as substrates for biologicals
Vol. 71: Utrecht, 1989	Monoclonal antibodies for therapy, prevention and *in vivo* diagnosis of human disease
Vol. 72: Annecy, 1989	Progress in animal retroviruses
Vol. 73: Shizuoka, 1990	Pertussis: Evaluation and research on acellular pertussis vaccines
Vol. 74: Bethesda, MD, 1990	Biological product freeze-drying and formulation
Vol. 75: London, 1990	Virological aspects of the safety of biological products
Vol. 76: Bethesda, MD, 1991	Continuous cell lines – Current issues
Vol. 77: Annecy, 1991	Standardization of the immunopharmacology of natural and synthetic immunomodulators
Vol. 78: Bethesda, MD, 1991	Poliovirus attenuation: Molecular mechanisms and practical aspects
Vol. 79: Ploufragan, 1992	The first steps towards an international harmonization of veterinary biologicals: 1993 and free circulation of vaccines within the E.E.C.
Vol. 80: Heidelberg, 1992	Transmissible spongiform encephalopathies-Impact on animal and human health.
Vol. 81: Cannes, 1992	Virological safety aspects of plasma derivatives.
Vol. 82: Albany, NY, 1993	Recombinant vectors in vaccine development.
Vol. 83: Annecy, 1993	Genetic stability and recombinant product consistency.
Vol. 84: Langen, 1993	Non-target effects of live vaccines.
Vol. 85: Santa Fee, NM, 1994	Genetics of streptococci, enterococci and lactococci.
Vol. 86: Langen, 1994	Replacement, reduction and refinement of animal experiments in the development and control of biological products.
Vol. 87: Geneva, 1995	New approaches to stabilisation of vaccines potency.
Vol. 88: Bethesda, MD, 1995	Viral safety and evaluation of viral clearance from biopharmaceutical products.
Vol. 89: Rome, 1995	Pertussis vaccine trials.
Vol. 90: Oslo, 1996	Fish vaccinology.
Vol. 91: San Francisco, CA, 1996	Development of specifications for biotechnology pharmaceutical products.
Vol. 92: Bergen, 1996	Modulation of the immune response to vaccine antigens.
Vol. 93: Annecy, 1996	Safety of biological products prepared from mammalian cell culture.
Vol. 94: Bethesda, MD, 1997	Simian virus 40 (SV40): a possible human polyomavirus.
Vol. 95: Paris, 1997	Preclinal and clinical development of new vaccines.
Vol. 96: Washington, DC, 1995	Characterization of biotechnology pharmaceutical products
Vol. 97: London, 1997	Biological characterization and assay of cytokines and growth factors.
Vol. 98: London, 1997	Inactivated influenza vaccines prepared in cell culture.
Vol. 99: Strasbourg, 1998	Animal sera, animal sera derivatives and substitutes used in the manufacture of pharmaceuticals: Viral safety and regulatory aspects.
Vol. 100: Geneva, 1998	A celebration of 50 years of progress in biological standardization and control at WHO.
Vol. 101: London, 1998	Alternatives to animals in the development and control of biological products for human and veterinary use.

Developments in Biologicals

Vol. 102: San Francisco, CA, 1999	Advances in transfusion safety.
Vol. 103: Annecy, 1999	Physico-chemical procedures for the characterization of vaccines.
Vol. 104: Langen, 1999	Development and clinical progress of DNA vaccines.
Vol. 105: Paris, 2000	Progress in polio eradication: vaccine strategies for the end game.
Vol. 106: Rockville, MD, 1999	Evolving scientific and regulatory perspectives on cell substrates for vaccine development.
Vol. 107: London, 2000	The design and analysis of potency assays for biotechnology products.
Vol. 108: Langen, 2001	Advances in transfusion safety - 2001.
Vol. 109: Washington, DC, 2000	Biologics 2000 – Comparability of biotechnology products.
Vol. 110: Palm Cove, 2001	Orphan Vaccines – Bridging the Gap.
Vol. 111: Utrecht, 2001	Advancing Science and Elimination of the Use of Laboratory Animals for Development and Control of Vaccines and Hormones.
Vol. 112: Bethesda, MD, 2001	Immunogenicity of Therapeutic Biological Products.
Vol. 113: Berlin, 2001	Process Validation for Manufacturing of Biologics and Biotechnology Products.
Vol. 114: Ames, IA, 2002	Vaccines for OIE List A and Emerging Animal Diseases
Vol. 115: Bergen, 2002	Laboratory Correlates of Immunity to Influenza – A Reassessment
Vol. 116: Los Angeles, CA, 2003	Development of Therapeutic Cancer Vaccines

IMPRIMERIE MEDECINE m+h HYGIENE
septembre-2004